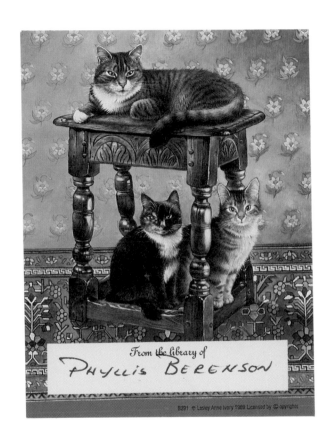

From the Library of

PHYLLIS BERENSON

B291 © Lesley Anne Ivory 1989 Licensed by © copyrights

I Am
Becoming the

Woman

I've Wanted

Other Anthologies by Sandra Haldeman Martz

When I Am an Old Woman I Shall Wear Purple

If I Had My Life to Live Over I Would Pick More Daisies

If I Had a Hammer: Women's Work in Poetry, Fiction, and Photographs

The Tie That Binds: A Collection of Writings about Fathers & Daughters/ Mothers & Sons

I Am
Becoming the
Woman
I've Wanted

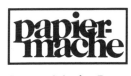

Papier-Mache Press
Watsonville, CA

First Edition

Cover art, "Blue Nude #2," © 1989 by Anna Price-Oneglia

Cover design by Cynthia Heier

Copyediting and editorial assistance by Shirley E. Coe

Typography by Prism Photographics

Library of Congress Cataloging-in-Publication Data

I am becoming the woman I've wanted / Sandra Haldeman Martz. — 1st ed.
    p.   cm.
  ISBN 0-918949-50-5 : $16.00.—ISBN 0-918949-49-1 (pbk.) : $10.00
  1. Women—Literary collections.   2. Body image—Literary collections.
3. Body, Human—Literary collections.   4. American literature—Women
authors.   5. American literature—20th century.
PS509.W6I13   1994
810.8'0352042—dc20   94-19650
                                                           CIP

For the women of *Atalanta, An Anthology of Creative Work Celebrating Women's Athletic Achievements*, with appreciation for their strength, courage, and inspiration.

Contents

Foreword

I Am Becoming the Woman I've Wanted grew out of my interest in looking at the ways in which our female physical attributes affect how we *are* in the world—how we see ourselves, how we act, how we interact with others—and how we are perceived by others which, in turn, affects how we are. This interplay of self and others reminds me of how, as a child, I would place two mirrors face to face, creating an endless succession of images where I would try, unsuccessfully, to discern where one left off and the next began. I grew up looking into those mirrors for something else I could not possibly find: perfection. Like many women, I spent years searching elsewhere for a sense of self-worth.

And so I wanted this collection to explore more than just women's body image or our conditioning to focus on being too much of one thing, too little of another. I hoped to find, as Victoria Wilgocki observed of contemporary women poets who write about the body, "a fierce and joyful reclaiming of what it is to be a woman in the landscape of a woman's body." As I read the almost four thousand submissions, I was not disappointed, although I did at times feel overwhelmed by the ambitiousness of this project. There was so much ground to cover, so many complexities. In the end, I chose material that reflected the breadth of the experiences that women had chosen to write about, selecting individual pieces that touched me personally or caused me to think about issues in new ways.

Much of the material about young women deals with anxiety and struggle: working through issues of self-image, feeling vulnerable, and sometimes being abused as a result of that vulnerability. As the narrators age, the stories and poems evolve toward a more empowered state as women claim their bodies and their power, challenging others' perceptions and ideas.

For adult women, motherhood emerges as an important motif: the emotional and physical intensity of the birth process, the devastation of miscarriage and infertility, or the choice to not have children. Women also wrote of physical differences—blindness, immobility, loss of hearing—or illnesses such as cancer, emphasizing the courage and strength found in their experiences.

Middle age—menopause and its accompanying hot flashes, soft bodies, wrinkles—is often welcomed and celebrated in the writings. And sexuality, along with a blossoming of creativity, comes into its own at midlife.

The poems and stories about old age are often filled with a delightful sense of humor and a comfortable acceptance of the physical changes that come with being very old. There is a clear message of wanting to meet death on one's own terms while having the support of loved ones in that last life experience.

Throughout this anthology, the writings are complemented by the work of some very talented photographers. These "visual poems" have much to say about the beauty and strength and wonder of women.

The diverse themes in this collection are tied together with the stunning title poem by Jayne Relaford Brown. Discovering "Finding Her Here" was one of the highlights of the selection process. After many, many readings I still cannot speak her words aloud without weeping. Her images touch me in ways that I can't explain. Is it the sensuousness of her "full moons" and "deep weathered baskets," or the way she acknowledges those years when life was hard, the survivorship? Maybe it is simply that I sense she too used to look in those mirrors. But what she now finds there informs and transforms our ideas of perfection, casting an affirming light on our paths toward self-love.

SANDRA HALDEMAN MARTZ

I Am
Becoming the

Woman

I've Wanted

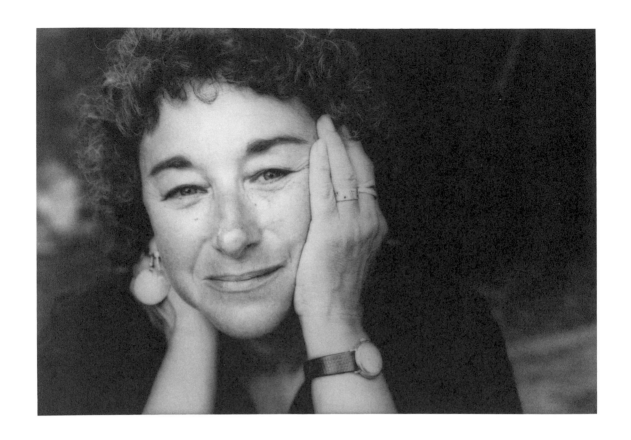

Finding Her Here

Jayne Relaford Brown

I am becoming the woman I've wanted,
grey at the temples,
soft body, delighted,
cracked up by life
with a laugh that's known bitter
but, past it, got better,
knows she's a survivor—
that whatever comes,
she can outlast it.
I am becoming a deep
      weathered basket.

I am becoming the woman I've longed for,
the motherly lover
with arms strong and tender,
the growing up daughter
who blushes surprises.
I am becoming full moons
      and sunrises.

I find her becoming,
this woman I've wanted,
who knows she'll encompass,
who knows she's sufficient,
knows where she's going
and travels with passion.
Who remembers she's precious,
but knows she's not scarce—
who knows she is plenty,
      plenty to share.

History of the Body

Linda Nemec Foster

For my daughter

Body within my body, I shape you out of almost nothing,
give you a tight envelope to surround your soul.
I deem you female—eyes cobalt blue, fingers long
and translucent—without even realizing it. And after
the quantum leap from single cell to complex organism,
much of your body's life is beyond my conscious thought:
your waking, your sleeping, the small objects of your
complete desire. Complete as the perfect wings
of the jay above your head or the pale stars that mark
your birth with nothing but pure light. Daughter,
I cannot give you anything so complete or perfect or pure.
But I can give you something better. Your body,
which is your life. And the fierce love of it that no one
can take away. And these words that will remind you
of that love. And your father's broad hand that opened
the door to it. And the blankness of the rest of this page
for your own words, your own history.

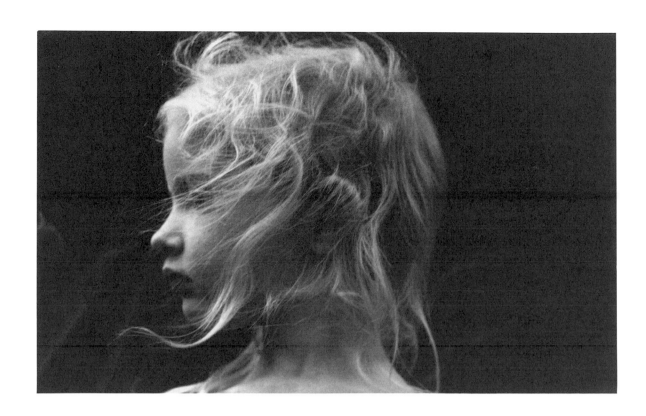

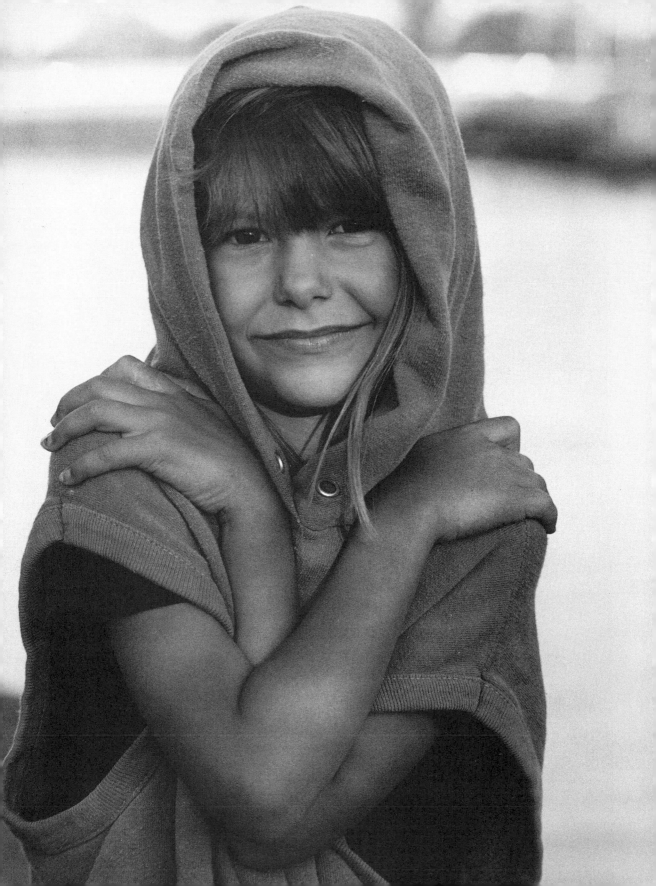

Applewood
Barbara Crooker

Out of the bare trees,
pink buds swell,
hold on and on
before they blush,
then blossom out,
unfolding to starry hearts,
transforming the orchard
in ruffles and lace,
lasting three days.

And our daughters too,
unfolding,
too large for swings,
too small for formals,
their pippin breasts,
their spindled limbs.

How slowly the apples grow,
taking rain inside,
wrapped in sun.
In August they look ripe,
but a taste puckers the tongue.
Not until storms and frost
will the sugar run.
For these young girls,
sneaking mascara,
sleeping with bunnies,
time is heavy and slow.

The apples hang on the boughs;
the weight, the weight
stretches the tree.
But these are the branches
that will not break;
the cycle that can't be broken.
These apples are full of juice and spirit,
a harvest of summer to savor all year.

And, mothers and daughters,
we'll end like Amish apple dolls,
wrinkled and dried,
turned into ourselves,
final
as red winesaps on the bough.

Room to Love

Jane Blue

An uncle, my grandmother's last child at home, occupies the sun porch suspended over the back garden. I do not remember his presence. My sister tells me he gave us our breakfast at the painted table in the kitchen, took us to the bathroom in the middle of the night. Daddy has gone off into the silence, and we have moved with Mother into Nana's house.

When my uncle marries, I inherit the room he has vacated, big paned windows facing both south and west, a little garden of nasturtiums and geraniums below, a view of rooftops all the way to the bay. An odd, narrow room with canvas on the floor, it becomes my nest, my haven.

I am four or five, and my life is changed forever because I have this room. My uncle's army cot becomes my bed; across from it there is a student desk and a dresser which Mother paints pink. They are crowded into a little nook by the tiny closet which juts into the room, added on sometime behind the closet in my sister's room. The room is not rectangular, but fits together in pieces like a puzzle. A low bookcase sits under the big windows at the foot of my bed. Mother has papered the walls with big flowers, painted the wood and the canvas of the floor green.

A mirror hangs above the dresser, hidden away behind the closet on a wall that is grooved, some odd and ancient paneling. I see different faces, different selves, when I look in the mirror, trying to decide who I am. This room is where I will live for the next seventeen years, but I always refer to it as my room in Nana's house.

I learn to love myself in solitude.

Nana never catches me, lying on my thin cot, exploring the places in my own body that give me a feeling of love. But when I prepare for confession with the help of a little black book, I decide that this is one of the sins of impurity: *impure thoughts or actions.*

"Alone or with others," the priest asks in his muffled, faceless voice.

"Alone," I answer. I do not know which is worse, but I suspect that it is my own sin, the sin of loving myself, alone.

Nana does discover my search for love once, obliquely, not head on.

But nothing was ever met head on.

My cousin, who is a year older than I, has come to our house to play, although no one really plays in Nana's house. His mother, my grandmother's oldest daughter, must have dropped him off, for she is not here. She would not leave us together for a moment, as she is the family guardian of morals.

Nana's rule has always been that if we have friends over, we must play in our rooms. We do not have friends, though, because Nana screens them carefully, and no one passes. Cousins are tolerated, as long as we go to my room. We are a girl and a boy, perhaps ten and eleven. My cousin has no sisters; I have no brothers. We are curious.

We decide to practice kissing. In high school, this cousin will have a reputation among the girls as a "good kisser," so I guess the practice was worthwhile.

What a nice feeling it is as we stand on the green, resilient canvas floor of my room; we are relaxed and warm, and find ourselves lying full length on my little bed, our bodies about the same size, pressed against each other's. I take off my glasses. We grow very, very quiet.

Nana's voice rises, disembodied, disorienting, from downstairs. She has been working in her study and is glad for the silence, but she looks up from her papers and realizes perhaps the extent of it, the vastness that rings into the quiet, loud as a gong.

"What are you two doing up there?"

We get up suddenly. I go to the mirror to straighten my hair.

"Nothing," I call downstairs in a shaky voice.

After this, I continue to try on selves in front of the mirror, but I do not touch myself, wake myself to myself; I am afraid to leave a mark like the one already on my soul, as they say in the catechism Nana makes sure I attend.

I wrap a white towel around my face to mimic the garb of a nun. I carve the initials of a boy into the grooved paneling. When I look in the mirror, a face stares back, grown and beautiful. I don't know who it belongs to.

I write poetry at my little desk, rushing to get the words down into a composition book with a sewn binding before the feeling passes, an ecstasy as I contemplate the view from my window on a balmy summer night, the full moon illuminating everything like liquid silver spread out on the world, or a silver curtain laid out to dry all the way to the bay.

I cannot describe how I feel any other way:

The moon shines on bushes and trees, it shines all around, it shines on the sea.

I remember these words all my life, and the magic of my solitary room comes back to me, and the magic of learning to love.

Fourteen

Pamela Ditchoff

She is the delicate and contained
pulse in my wrist, an insistent and tender
reminder of my mortality. My daughter at fourteen shines
like a mirror through skin close to her bones,
drawn smooth and tight with hope;
she is a song I sing with grace.

I watch as she bends her neck to contain the tender
oboe reed between her lips, and I touch each round,
shining bone, tuning my hopes to her grace note.

Photo by Therese Becker

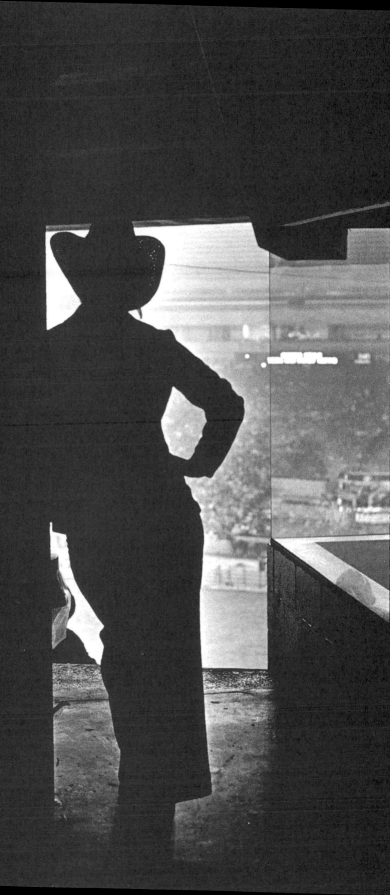

Foot Loose

Deborah Shouse

I fiddle with my purse as I stand outside the dressing room, waiting for my daughter Sarah to try on five bathing suits. A small boy crawls out from under the swinging door of a nearby stall, then moves into the empty room beside me. I'd like to crawl after him. This is my third dressing room this evening, and I need some diversion.

"I'm fat!" Sarah wails.

"You have a nice body," I say.

"You have to say that. You're my mother."

I sink onto the floor, stretching my legs across the aisle. I pluck a pin from the floor and notice Sarah's feet, long and surprisingly elegant. These slender feet and ankles could belong to any woman. A princess, a loan officer, a midnight blues singer, a love-struck poet. They could belong to a cousin or sister or mother. But they belong to my daughter, and they once lived inside me.

Sarah opens the dressing room door and gives me a glimpse of a bright yellow-and-pink suit, high cut in the legs, low cut in the back. I am shocked by her sophisticated beauty. My moody thirteen-year-old looks like a Club Med ad.

"My thighs are disgusting," she says, closing the door.

"You look wonderful," I say.

I remember the summer evenings when I sat in night school, Sarah large and ripe in my stomach. I was the only student in the M.B.A. program who carried a pillow underneath her managerial accounting text. In the unair-conditioned classroom, sticky with heat and tired from the day's work, I struggled to find a spot my body approved of. My belly pressed against the confines of the desk. While the teacher discussed accounting strategies, my baby stirred. Feisty feet kicked me, reminding me of things that cannot be calculated.

"I can't get these suits hung up," Sarah says and throws out a pile of suits and their hangers. I sit on the floor and attach each suit to its hanger. The boy makes a cat sound as he crawls back down the aisle.

"Get off that floor," a harsh voice commands. I almost leap up, but remember, in my family, I am now that voice.

Sarah slips on her clothes and buries her feet in disreputable black tennis shoes. I remember when her soft baby feet had nothing to do with the floor or dirt. They were made for kicking, kissing, and holding. Those innocent baby toes didn't know about cross-training shoes, matching socks, panty hose, and heels.

"I might like this one." Sarah emerges, holding the yellow and pink suit. "But I can't decide."

"I'm getting tired," I say as we leave the dressing room. The bright bang of MTV music and loud splash of the neon T-shirts hits me as we stroll through the Juniors section. I dream of the women's department where clothes are muted, tame, less frenetic.

"One more store, just one more. I'll hurry, I promise. Please?" Sarah gives me her best-daughter-in-the-world smile.

"All right. One more store," I agree.

Thirty minutes, three racks, and ten suits later, I sit outside the dressing room again. I brush my hair and watch Sarah's feet drift in and out of suits. I remember the family outing we made to buy her first shoes. I struggled to cram her curling foot into that impossibly small white shoe.

Sarah steps into a suit and kicks her tennis shoes out of the way. When she was young, she sat for hours, tying and untying tennis shoes. She knotted them together, then called me for help in getting them undone.

She turns now, probably examining herself in the mirrors. Her feet are poised, like a dancer's. I remember her first patent leather dress-up shoes with the shiny tops and the slick soles.

"I think this is the one," she says, modeling briefly a striped navy blue suit.

"Is it comfortable? Can you bend over? Will it stay on when you jump off the board?" I ask.

"Oh, mother," Sarah says.

"Oh, mother, let me play in your shoes," she used to say. She clomped around in my heels, then scuttled around in my sandals. Now, her feet are longer than mine. She is a Cinderella too strong and real for glass slippers.

She dresses and we pay for the suit. Naturally she has selected the only swimming apparel in the western hemisphere that is not on sale.

Sarah's shoelaces flop as we walk out of the store. I know better than to suggest she tie them. The feet that kicked inside me, the feet that begged to be played with, that hurried to me when I came home from work, the tired little feet that pleaded to be carried, can outrun me now.

"Thanks for the suit," Sarah says, as we stride briskly through the mall. We have a few more minutes before we reach the car and she sinks into the radio station and far away from me. A few minutes before she plants her feet indolently on the dash and I set mine firmly on the accelerator and brake. A few more minutes when our steps are evenly matched and we are walking comfortably, like two friends.

Ceremony

Suellen Wedmore

I chased red-winged blackbirds
across Illinois fields, laughed as I climbed sycamore trees,
and sometimes in the twilight, I believed
I would not change.
Until one night my breasts swelled

and hair came in moist and secret places,
and my legs and arms
unfolded. I ran with awkward steps, drumming emotion,
and when the bleeding came, I was afraid. I wanted
to be painted in red earth like the Cheyenne,

bathe in chamomile, hide in the sweet-grass smell
of the moon lodge with my kind grandmother
until the defiling passed. On a night

of a waxing moon I coughed, and when my father
rubbed medicine across my chest, he saw
the changing. A Cheyenne father marks the time
with the gift of a horse. I looked up
as my father stepped away from me,

saw the softening of his eyes.

Butchering Time

Carol Newman

Cora felt dizzy, but she couldn't fall. She was already lying flat. Tall blades of prairie grass whipped around her in the hot Oklahoma wind. She squinted into the cloudless blue. Maybe she could float. If what had just happened was possible, then perhaps it was possible to drift away into the distant sky.

That morning, as usual, she had risen at first light and built a fire in the dusty clearing outside the sod cabin. She boiled coffee, baked biscuits in a black Dutch oven, fried potatoes in a deep skillet, and made gravy.

As if drawn by the mingling smells, her father and two brothers shuffled out and squatted in the dust to eat. She handed a tin plate to her father, then one to Ben and one to Willie. "Mornin', Papa."

Just as he had never replied when Cora's mother spoke to him, he did not reply now. With thin red hair and pale skin, Papa still looked more like a coal miner than a farmer, even after two years away from Ohio.

Ben and Willie scraped their plates and also said nothing. Willie was nearly sixteen, and Cora knew it made him mad that she was almost as tall as he was. Ben was only thirteen, a year younger than Cora. Sometimes when Cora saw Papa watching her she worked extra hard. But strength or age didn't matter; they were menfolk and ate first.

Inside the cabin, baby Esther began crying. Every morning since their mother died of flu, Esther awoke calling, "Mamamama."

Esther stood on the bed she shared with Cora, rubbing her fists in her thick curly hair. Smoothing the dark ringlets back from the baby's teary face, Cora thought of how her mother used to brush her hair.

"Better enjoy this hair, girl. It's probably the only gold you'll ever see." Sometimes when Mama was brushing Cora's hair she would put down the brush and forget to pick it up, stroking the long straight hair with her hand before dividing it and plaiting it into two long braids. What would Mama think if she saw the way Cora wore her hair loose on her back now?

Cora held out her hand. "Now Esther, you could just get yourself off this bed instead of crying. You come on outside if you're so hungry. I have a biscuit and gravy for you."

Cora lifted Esther to her hip. Three plates sat in the dust. "Looks like Papa and the boys have already gone to the field. You sit on the log, and I'll get our breakfast."

After they had eaten, Cora scooped dirt and put it over the fire, stirring the ashes with a stick until she was sure every ember was dead. Dry prairie grass stretched for miles around the cabin. "Watch that fire, woman," Papa had told Mama. "This grass catches fire, we'll all be goners."

Cora tied the leftover biscuits and potatoes with some salted meat in a feed sack, washed the plates, and left them inside on the table. With Esther tucked on her hip, the men's work shirts bundled under her other arm, and a piece of her mother's lye soap clutched in her hand, Cora pretended to be a pony and galloped with Esther to the creek.

With its trees and mossy banks, the creek reminded Cora of Ohio. It was her favorite place in this flat country which left her eyes hungry for the sight of woods and hills. Where the bank sloped down to a shallow pool, Cora knelt on a flat, red rock. Esther, safe from the deeper water, sat at the edge of the rock swinging her legs.

"Here, hold the soap for me. No, don't put it in the water. I want it to last." Cora dipped the collar of Papa's shirt into the water. "And don't put that in your mouth. It's got lye in it."

Last winter, Ben and Willie had held one of the hogs while Papa cut its throat. The animal's one scream had hung in the air with its frosty breath.

When the men finished butchering, Cora's mother built up the fire for soap making. "Look here, Cora. Now you help me do this. You're going to make good soap."

The boiling fat and lye made Cora feel sick. "I will Mama, but I hear the baby crying. Maybe I best feed her first."

Cora had escaped the soap making that time, but this year her father would expect her to do it. She wished she could make the soap last.

She spread the shirts on the grass to dry where the wind sent little shivers down the sleeves.

Back at the cabin, Cora carried water and food to the chickens. The hens clucked noisily around the girls' feet, and Esther backed away as the chickens moved closer. When Esther was about to cry, Cora scooped her up, away from the pecking birds, and headed for the garden.

While Cora pulled weeds from long, dusty rows of vegetables, Esther stumbled along the rough ground. Finally Cora said, "Well, that's enough of that. My back hurts. Anyway, it's time to take the men their meal. Come on, Esther. Let's go to the field."

Taking the cloth-wrapped food and pail of water and dipper, they started across the prairie to where the men were working. The sun hung overhead, beating on the blowing grass.

In the distance, Cora saw her father bending to lift something onto the wagon. Then he straightened and looked toward the girls coming across the prairie.

"Call to Papa, Esther. Say 'Pa-pa.'"

"Puh, puh," Esther said and bounced up and down on Cora's hip.

"I think he heard you. He's looking this way." The hot wind swirled the fabric of her dress.

Cora turned her face into the wind, and her long hair streamed back. Her dress billowed behind her. "Look, Esther. We're sailboats."

When they reached the men, Papa said, "We need fresh water."

For the first time, Cora noticed Papa's teeth; they were small and sort of brown around the edges. She wasn't sure she had ever seen them before, but today Papa was smiling.

"Cora, go to the creek and fetch some more water."

"Yes, Papa." She set the food in the wagon and plopped Esther beside it.

Papa leaned against the wagon and chewed his meat and biscuit. Ben and Willie grabbed for what was left. Cora picked up an empty pail and started toward the creek. She had almost reached the trees along the water when she heard him behind her.

"You're the woman now," he said.

At first Cora couldn't understand what he was saying. Papa grabbed her around the waist, and she struggled to keep her balance. Dust rose up. She tried to scramble away, but he pushed her down, shoving her dress up to her chest and yanking the tie loose at the waist of her cotton underwear.

Cora had seen the livestock mate, and she knew men and women did the same, but she couldn't believe what was happening. As he straddled Cora and opened his overalls, she thought of the wild stallion that had broken into the little corral where they kept the plow horse, Dolly. The stallion, walleyed with wildness, had reared and come down on Dolly's rump, hooves slashing at her withers. Dolly's whinnies had sounded like crying. Cora ran away and hid in the brush until her mother called, "Cora, you come here. There's chores need doing."

But this time she couldn't run away. Papa loomed over her. She closed her eyes, embarrassed for him to see her nakedness. With one knee he pushed apart her thighs. Then there was pain and wet and the words in her head as she silently pleaded, *Papa, no, oh stop, please stop, Papa.*

And then, almost as if he had heard her, he did stop.

He stood and buttoned his overalls. "You bring that water, hear." And he ambled away in the direction of the field.

She remained for a while as he had left her, lying in the prairie grass, looking at the sky and praying to be taken away. At last she gave up, and like a sleepwalker on the longest night of the year, shuffled to the cabin.

After a while, Cora returned to the creek, carrying a piece of her mother's lye soap. She stood in deep water until her dress was wet and heavy, then she undressed. Her two thin garments sank to the sharp rocks on the bottom. Slowly she washed her body, dipping time and time again into the water.

No need to be careful of the hard, yellow soap. She would make more at butchering time.

Womansong

Marilyn Johnson

Maybe it begins the day you pledge allegiance,
face the flag and suddenly clutch your left clavicle
because you find a tender puff of breast
where yesterday your heart was

Or maybe it happens later when you're walking home
from school and they rush you on the street—
those boys who reach out fast, disgrace your blouse
with rubs of dirt, their laughter
stinging hot against your face.
And you bite your rage, swallow your tears
because the fact is, your territory's up for grabs
and somehow it's your own damned fault.

And one day you stand at your mirror
armed with jars and razor blades against the scents
and grasses of your shameless bleeding body,
and you see what you've become—a freak
manufactured to disguise the real one,
the one who sometimes still recalls your innocence,
the time before you became a dirty joke.

And maybe it begins to end the day
you try against the odds to love yourself again.
Even though you know the worst thing
you can call someone is cunt,
you try to love that flesh and fur you are,
that convoluted, prehistoric flower,
petals dripping weeds and echoing
vaguely fragrant odors of the sea.

A Place to Rest

Chris Mandell

Then, she could stomach anything:
endless binges,
day and night,
anything sugary, or whatever,
anything at all to stretch
her stomach to the limit,
that limit
at the end of emptiness
that place (her *own* place) of
absolutely NO
more.
It was like a wall
she could rest against a moment
(she lived for this moment)
before heaving it all up
and starting again.
Then, the hunger was a terror in her gut.

Now, the hunger is an anger
compacted in the small squares
of her teeth,
fierce and specific:
thick marrow of crunched chicken bones,
white protective pulp of orange,
woody core of pineapple,
canned salmon vertebrae.
For a treat, she buys five cans of salmon,
eats five sets of vertebrae,
and leaves the meat.

These foods puzzle others,
but not her,
since she feels definitely,
day and night,
the lines of her body thicken,
embracing the precise shape
she now rests in.

Everything That Falls Has Wings

Kathy M. Parkman

I write the truth and I write lies. Mostly I write lies. For instance: *I am happy when I'm with a lot of people.* And this is a lie: *I am secure with the way I look.* These are lies I write for Karina, my therapist. She says she wants to help me.

In the journal that only I see, I write the truth. The truth is I am hopeless. I don't feel this way all of the time. Sometimes I am happy, or at least I make myself think that I am happy. Taylor makes me happy. The therapist was his idea. He is worried about me. He says he worries constantly.

My clothes are big and dark. "What are you afraid of?" Karina asks.

"Afraid of?" I am staring at the painting behind her. I always stare at it when I should be looking at her. It is a bright painting of a woman sitting in a yellow chair with an orange cat on her lap. The woman's hair is so long that it drapes over the arm of the chair.

"You hide under those big clothes."

"I like my clothes."

"Because you can hide in them?" Karina is not smiling. She doesn't smile very often in this office. But once I saw her at a restaurant with a man and she was laughing, and he was feeding her shrimp. She did not see me.

"My clothes serve their purpose, just like yours do."

She shifts in her chair and fires her next question, "How are things between you and Taylor?"

"OK. He worries about me too much."

"And why do you think he worries about you?"

"Same old thing, you know."

"Tell me, Rachel. Tell me why."

I don't have to tell her why. She knows. She looks at her watch.

"Time to go?" I say.

"Just about. I want you to continue your journal for me and bring it in next week. Try to write more about what you're feeling."

On my way out the receptionist gives me the bill to give to Taylor. The envelope is always sealed. I have no idea how much he pays for these sessions.

I drive home in the rain and imagine myself veering to the left and colliding with the cars coming toward me. I imagine every element of the crash: the solid impact, the folding in of the front end, the continued crumpling until the front window meets the back one and I am caught between. I see it all in slow motion. I see myself throwing my hands up in surrender, knowing it's all over. I never see any more of it—the ambulance, the blood, the police notifying my family. My vision doesn't reach those scenes.

I live alone. I've lived alone for three years, ever since I returned from a trek through Europe. As soon as I got back I knew that I could no longer stand living in my parents' house. I need privacy and freedom. My parents worry about me, too. They blame themselves for my problem.

The problem is this: I am starving. At least that is what everyone tells me. I don't feel like I am starving. I am not hungry, ever. Food disgusts me. If I am forced to eat I will immediately vomit; it is an involuntary action. These are the things I will consume on my own: lettuce, water, coffee, zucchini, tomato juice, and, occasionally, an apple. In Europe I ate bread, but I won't eat it here. There it was a matter of survival.

Taylor likes to take me out for dinner. I always order salad, and this upsets him. He's learned that I will eat more if I'm drunk. He's tricked me with wine a few times, but it doesn't work anymore. I am smarter than he is. He is coming over tonight.

The doorbell rings, and I look through the peephole. There is Taylor all warped and big-headed. He looks like a caricature, and it makes me laugh.

"What's so funny?" he asks when I open the door.

"You," I say and kiss him. "You through that peephole."

"Not fair," he says. "How was your session?"

"Same as always. Karina asks stupid questions. The bill is on my desk."

He picks it up and puts it in the inside pocket of his jacket. "What do you want to do tonight?"

"How about a movie?"

"What kind of movie?" He rests his hands on my shoulders and looks straight into my eyes. His eyes are blue with green shooting through them like shards of glass. His are the most magnificent eyes I have ever seen. I think that is why I fell in love with him so quickly.

"We can see whatever's playing down at Tower."

The sun disappears as we walk down the street. I get a chill so Taylor puts his arm around me and pulls me into him. He is older than I am. I met him right after his fiancée called off their wedding and moved to Spain to model. He was a wreck for a while, but now they're friends. Her name is Tasha, and I met her once. She was home for her sister's graduation or something, and she agreed to meet us at a café. I didn't know exactly what she looked like because Taylor burned all the photographs of her, except for one of them in France, and she was blurry from moving to swat at a bee. We waited for her for over an hour. We waited, and Taylor ate bits of cheese while I held his hand. Finally she came through the door, and there she was: almost six feet tall, blond, wearing a leopard print coat, a leather miniskirt, black sling-backs, gloves, and sunglasses. She kissed Taylor on both cheeks and shook my hand. I looked down at my big brown sweater, my jeans, and I wanted to cry. Taylor told me later that Tasha said I was beautiful but much, much too thin.

"Hmm. *Wings of Desire* again," Taylor says as soon as he can see the marquee.

"Good. My favorite."

There are only a few people in the theater, and I am glad. It is a beautiful place, built in the 1920s and recently restored. The walls have paintings of nude women draped in sheer cloth, each surrounded by a thick gilded frame. The women are all gazing upward, and not one of them is smiling. The seats are covered with deep red velvet, and the carpet has a wild floral pattern. This is a peaceful place. This is a place for escape.

The movie makes me cry again, though I tried not to this time. The angels in the library get me every time. When I was in Berlin I went to that library and just sat there for hours. I tried to sense anything out of the ordinary, but nothing happened.

On our way home we pass the pub where I used to work. Taylor says, "Wanna get a drink?"

And I really do feel like having a drink. Karina will want to know exactly *why* I felt like having a drink, and I will write this: *I wanted to have a drink because the movie made me feel empty. I wanted to fill part of the space with wine. I wanted wine so that I could fill the rest of the space with sex.* I will write this because it is what she will think anyway. She asked me once if I had lost my sex drive.

"I don't think so," I said. But the truth is that I rarely want to have sex.

I do it for Taylor, and if I have some wine I do it for myself, too.

We sit at a corner table and hold hands.

The waitress comes over to us. "Rachel. Hi. I haven't seen you around lately." Her name is Lorna, and she's bulimic. She talked me into going to a few twelve-step meetings with her last year, but they were too depressing. I only went to three, and I never talked.

"Hi, Lorna. Have you met Taylor?"

He shakes her hand. "Nice to meet you. We want wine." He smiles, and I excuse myself to the rest room.

Lorna comes in after me. "Hey," she says. "How are you doing?"

"I'm OK. How about you?"

She seems shaky, agitated. "I'm doing all right. Good days, bad days. This new bartender hooked me up with some speed. It helps to keep things under control, you know?"

"Be careful with that stuff."

"So this Taylor guy seems pretty cool. Been seeing him long?"

"Almost a year. He's paying for me to see this therapist. It's kind of weird. Makes me feel crazy."

"You're not crazy. You're just afraid of getting fat. You're just afraid, like all of us. You are pretty thin though. A lot thinner than before, I can see it in your face."

"I think I'm about the same. You just haven't seen me in a while."

She takes a tiny envelope out of her apron pocket and shakes two tablets into her palm. "The magic pills," she says and swallows them. "Back to work!"

The door swings closed behind her, and I look at myself in the mirror. I repowder the dark circles under my eyes, pinch my cheeks, and go back out to Taylor.

"I love you," I say to him before I even sit down. "Let's drink this wine."

We are both a little drunk as we walk home, and it starts to rain again. Taylor puts his jacket over our heads, and we stand in the middle of the street, kissing.

"Will you make love with me tonight?" he asks.

"I would love to make love with you tonight," I say, and breathe in the rain, and him, and the scent of wine on our tongues.

My apartment is warm. We take off our wet clothes and stand by the wall heater. While the front of my body warms up, Taylor stands behind me and combs my hair. I get a little chill each time the comb reaches the ends and a drop of water falls on my back and rolls down my spine. He lifts my hair from my neck and kisses me behind the ear.

"Ooh, the magic spot," I say and turn to face him.

"Yes," he says, pulling me closer, "magic."

I dream that I am in my apartment, and I find a door I didn't know was there. I open it and find a room with high ceilings and no windows. There is a huge fish-bowl filled with animal skins. I take one out and tear at the remaining flesh with my teeth. Blood drips down the sides of my mouth, and I keep chewing at the flesh.

Taylor is putting his pants on when I wake up.

"What time is it?" I ask him.

"A little after seven. I have to get to work. I'll call you after my shift."

He does the morning classical show at the public radio station. It is called "Clearly Classical," and he is "Your host, Taylor Vaughn." Sometimes people recognize his name and say, "Hey, you're on the radio," as if he didn't know. I like it when that happens, and I think Taylor does, too.

"OK, baby," I say and walk him to the door. "I meet with Dr. Anton today, and I'll be home about two."

I finished college last year, but I'm doing an independent study with my favorite professor. Dr. Anton wants me to call him Jeff, but it doesn't seem right, even though we meet at his house. I love his house. It is the only real Victorian in town, and he and his wife swear it's haunted. His office is set up in the parlor which has its own entrance from the front porch. His two red Abyssinians sleep in the window and think they own the world. We meet to discuss poetry, but we usually talk about our dreams.

"Rachel, come in." Dr. Anton always greets me this way, almost as if he wasn't expecting me.

"Hi." I put my big coat over the back of the chair. "How's the book going?"

"I finished chapter six just this morning. I'm going to take a break from it before I start the stuff on Bly. But that's all boring, how are you?"

"I'm OK."

"You look a little tired." One of the princess cats jumps down from the windowsill and climbs on his lap. "Want some coffee?"

"No, thanks. I had a little too much to drink last night and stayed up late." I smile without thinking.

"Oh. Good night, huh?" He takes a bag from his desk and opens it. "Fig bar?"

"No, I'm fine. I had this dream."

"OK, tell me about it. Poetry can always wait." He leans forward a little and strokes the cat in perfect rhythm.

I tell him about the dream, about how I could almost taste the rotting flesh, how I could feel the fur and skin caught in my teeth.

"Can I get some water?" I ask when I am finished.

"Of course," he smiles.

I walk through the front room and the living room to get to the kitchen. There is a Casanova chair that I have never seen before. It is covered in red velvet like the chairs at Tower Theater. I want to sit in one of the S's curves, but I am afraid of such an antique. I am also afraid that Dr. Anton's wife might be home and catch me. I've never seen her directly, I have only caught glimpses of her moving from one room to another, like a ghost. I tiptoe, but the floor creaks anyway. I could never be alone in this house. I pour a glass of water from a heavy pitcher and walk quickly back to the parlor.

"Nice chair," I say when I get back.

"The Casanova? Had to fight like a dog at the auction to get that one. It was worth it though. The cats love it."

"So, poetry?"

"Rachel, I want to talk to you about something else. I've had you in classes for four years now, right?"

"Yeah. Geez, four years."

"And during that time you've changed. You've become thinner and thinner."

"Oh, god, not you, too."

"Yes, me, too. I know you're seeing a therapist, but have you been to a doctor?"

"Yeah, about a year ago. He told me I just need to eat more."

"Great." He pulls his chair up close to mine and touches my hand. "I am worried about you."

"Well, you know, everyone is worried about me. Take a number."

"Don't let this get you, Rachel. Don't give it that much power."

"I think I'm going to go now. I want to be alone." I stand up and get my coat. Dr. Anton writes something down on a little card.

"Here," he says and hands it to me. "This woman is a friend of mine. She's a doctor. She can help you. Call her, OK?"

At a red light I take the card out of my pocket and stare at it. *Claire Maxwell.* Claire wants to help me, too. Dr. Anton is probably calling her right now to tell her that one of his students might call. "Her name is Rachel, and she needs help," he will say. Then they will laugh about something and talk about normal things.

I drive fast to get to Taylor's apartment. He should be there. There is someone else on the radio now. I see his car and know I am in luck.

His studio is one of my favorite places. It is what I want my place to look like, but I'm too neat. I live better in starkness. He has tapestries and huge pieces of fabric covering the walls. There are plants on every table and windowsill and on the floor. His books and tapes and CDs spill from the shelves and are all over the rug in little piles.

"It's so good to see you," I say and put my arms around him. He smells like garlic. "Cooking?"

"Pesto. It's almost ready. I was going to call you later. It's only one; did you meet with Dr. Anton?"

"Yeah, I left early." I follow him over to his little corner kitchen and watch him stir. He takes down bottles from his spice rack and shakes them into the pot of green.

"Everything OK?" He holds the spoon up to my mouth so I can taste. I stick my tongue out and barely touch it to the sauce.

"Good. Yeah, everything's OK. You know, I've been learning from him for four years. That's a long time, four years."

"Are you sure you're OK?"

"I'm sure. Can I lie down for a while?"

I fall asleep remembering a book I read about a group of people who survived for years by photosynthesis and one thin wafer a day. It was possible because they believed it. When I was weaning myself from food I kept remembering those people, believing that I, too, could live solely by the sun.

I sleep for hours, and when I wake up Taylor is kneeling by the bed looking at me. He has been crying.

Karina calls me on the day of our session and tells me to wear a leotard or a bathing suit under my clothes. She wants to do a body tracing so that I can see my true size. I tell her no, but she persists.

I dig through my dresser drawers to find my old ballet stuff. I haven't danced in years, and I'm afraid it will all be too small. I pull on the black tights and the burgundy leotard with the low back. It's baggy, and I am surprised. I stand in front of the long mirror on the back of my bedroom door and look at myself in perfect first position. I try second, move into third, raise one arm above my head and stretch my neck. This is what my dance instructors always wanted me to look like. I was too heavy then, too slow and grounded. Now I could fly.

Over the leotard and tights I put on a dark grey sweater, black sweatpants, and an army jacket.

I walk into Karina's office and there is butcher paper on the floor.

"Let's do the tracing first," she says. "I'll leave while you get undressed. Just open the door when you're ready."

I pull off my big clothes and leave them in a heap on the floor. I open the door and lie down on the paper.

"OK," Karina says, standing above me with a magic marker. "I'm just going to trace around your body with this pen, and then you can put your clothes back on."

I close my eyes as she follows the lines of my body. She doesn't trace around each finger, but instead draws around them, making them into mittens.

"All finished," she says as the pen reaches the top of my head again. "You can get dressed."

I stand up and look at what she's done. It's like a police chalk drawing of where a dead body was found. It is a tiny body, a child's body, but tall. Karina brings out a mirror from a closet. "Look at yourself in here," she says, "and then look at the tracing."

"Yeah?" I look from one to the other.

"Do you see the same thing?"

"No. Here I see me, and there I see paper."

"What about the size?"

"The body on the paper is tiny."

"It's your body, Rachel. That is your tiny body."

"It only looks so small because it's down there on the ground," I say. She tapes it to the wall.

"There. Now what?" she says.

"It's still tiny," I say. "Take it down. I don't want to look at it anymore. Take it down." I realize I am yelling. I sit down in the chair and start to cry.

I can't stop crying, so Karina calls Taylor to come and get me. "You should just go home and rest," Karina says and touches my shoulder. It is the first time she has touched me. "Here are your clothes. Taylor will be here soon."

I cry for the entire drive across town, and once we are inside my apartment Taylor lies down with me in my bed and holds me until I fall asleep.

"It hurts so much." These are the first words I say when I wake up. "It hurts so much."

I call Dr. Claire Maxwell's office to make an appointment. The receptionist tells me to come this afternoon. I try to think of an excuse to make it another day, but I find myself saying, "OK, today at two will be fine."

I decide to take a shower for the event. I run my hands over my body, feeling the hardness of the bones right beneath my skin. I go over each rib, counting them, and up to my collarbones. My breasts have kept a little of their softness.

I stand wet and naked in front of my mirror and push my stomach out as far as I can. It doesn't bulge, but instead comes out even to my ribs. I squint at my image to see the outline of myself, then I focus. Squint, focus. I wrap my robe around me and take a nap.

The waiting room is decorated in shades of grey with deep rose chairs to match the picture frames that hold black-and-white photographs of flowers. I am alone looking at one of a calla lily when a woman appears behind me.

"Do you like the photos?" she asks.

"I love them."

"I took them. I'm Claire." She shakes my hand and smiles. She is beautiful. "You're Rachel, right?"

"Yes. Dr. Anton gave me your name."

"I know. He called me. Come into my office."

I follow her down the hall that is lined with more of her photographs, more black-and-white flowers. In the office she sits next to me on a grey couch.

"Today I want to just check you out, take some blood, run a few tests, do an electrolyte workup, see how things are going in your body."

"OK."

"Rachel, how do you feel?"

"You sound like my therapist."

"No, *physically*, how do you feel?"

"Pretty good most of the time. A little tired."

"Do you know how much you weigh?"

"No. I haven't weighed myself for about two years. It was at a drug store in Paris, and I was forty-two kilos."

"Forty-two kilos. That's about ninety-two pounds. Do you want to see how much you weigh now?"

"All right," I say and walk with her to the scale. "Should I take my boots off?"

"If you want to."

I take them off, step on the scale, and close my eyes. I hear Claire moving the weight, but I don't know if it's going up or down.

"An even eighty," she says.

"Eighty?" I can hardly say the word.

"Let's sit down," she says, and we do. She holds both of my hands. "I'm not going to lie to you, Rachel. If we don't get some weight on you, you're going to have to go into the hospital. Your body is in starvation mode, and it's allowing you to function, but that won't last forever. It's kind of in denial about the situation right now, but at some point it will shut down."

"Will I die?"

"We need to get some weight on you. It's not going to be easy. I know it's frightening to think about eating, but we'll take it slow."

"Will you help me?"

"Of course I will help you, Rachel. Of course."

On my way out Claire stops me. "Wait," she says, and takes the calla lily photo down. "I want you to have this one."

I look at her, at the blank spot on the wall, take the lily from her hands, and say, "Thank you. Thank you so much."

I write the truth and I write lies. This is the truth: I look in the mirror now and see what others see. I am only half here, and I don't know where I've gone.

The Fat Lady Speaks

Joanne McCarthy

Fat is my fortress. It
keeps you from me. I
prize this great body, its
fierce implacable strength.

For I move when I choose to.
You cannot force me.
Wherever I go I mock
weakness and famine. Stare
if you will. You
are afraid of me.

Men pale at my
hunger. They are not men
with me. And women
shrink away, scorn
in their narrow eyes
but I despise them. They
bend to the will of others.
I do not bend at all.

I am a mighty goddess
a prehistoric queen
symbol of wealth and
terrible power.
Trifle with me
and I will
crush
you.

Rhonda, from the Runway at Diamond Don's

Liz Abrams-Morley

I'd love lights that blind. The girls
on stage at J.T.'s Place pull
plastic cherries from their crotches,
toss them out to hands and leering
faces that they never see, footlights
so bright they're a curtain
pulled between the leer and leered
at. Here in the sticks, out State

Route 53, the boss won't spring
for dazzle. I work this crowd
to cowboy music scratched
from a Motorola and wear purple
vinyl boots to gallop plywood—fifty
bucks a night for three, three-
minute gigs. Pays the rent; the drinks
I get for free. College boys

come Friday nights, ten to a car, heard
girls here put themselves through hell
and school on tips. I got a tip
it doesn't take a Ph.D. to figure; Don
started that one. Here, we learn
by doing, watch
that yellow line Don painted on
the runway so his girls would know

exactly what part of the show to show
what part. It's measured; tops
fall after eight. Bottoms: twist

your butt, gyrate on five, pluck
hook from eye so buckskin mini falls,
under it all, my gun tucked in G-string.

I draw on two, dance
buck naked for exactly eight brief
bouncing beats; it sure beats
serving highballs to the regulars who
always want talk and there's not one
thought in their goddamned pouchy faces.

I can make my face like that, dead
on the count of three, when I burst
from behind the yellow curtain. I empty
my brain, eyes, even my cheeks
don't shimmy when I shimmy my god-
given. I used to want to see
who came to see me dance. Two coeds
in floor-length nightgowns once parked

themselves, front and center like
they watched some high class fashion
show, made fashion showy noises, too:
*That one has saggy boobs. The ass
on that one's bony,* as if they thought
to try us on, buy one in each spring
color. Mother's Day eve, two years
past, it was six polyester plaid type
men, bald, and not a one with face

hair, or expressions for that matter.
Brought matching wives, I swear-to-god,
those ladies smelled like
Ida's Beauty Shoppe and each was pinned
with a rose corsage. Their men
called them "Mommy." *Mommy would like
a sloe-gin fizz. Mommy needs you to move
so she can watch the show, Miss.*

The mommies never said shit, or
*Jesus Christ will you look at the tits
on that one, Maude.* When I get old
no farmer's going to cut my vocal
chords, load me on a truck
and truck me off to celebrate my child-
bearing years with beers and naked
dancers here in the asshole

of Dane County. Faces
out there, I don't bother
with anymore. What's going to top
twelve blank old folks in church
clothes anyway, I tell the new
girls. I could teach them tricks,

could teach a college course on
going blank and Don would thank me
for it. You burn too much
energy smiling in the eyes of all

those guys you thought had come
for a moment with you, Rhonda Rodeo
Cowgirl Princess. Call me a down-
beat, Miss Dee

Pressed. I'm just
a pro. After a few acts
I didn't have to count to know
when to drop what. It's all measured
here—beats, gin, even Don's
lopsided grin when he hands you
fifty and a robe.

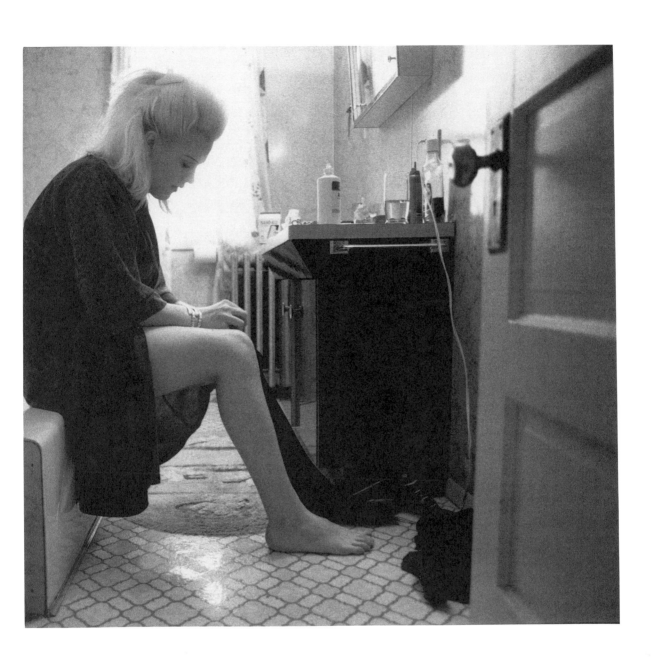

Shadow Brush

Judith Infante

I hesitate to name the woman
who sleeps behind my bed. A few layers
of board and plaster between us, we each live
alone—I with stacks of books, she with nightly
men. I hear them, inches from my deconstructed
novel, inside worrisome dreams; they rock and slam,
they shake the walls, spackle dust on my headboard.

Mornings I drink tea, write thin lines, imagine
that she washes glasses, changes the sheets.
Perhaps she also ponders half-familiar
photographs. Across her balcony might drift
tears of paper, wadded-up thoughts, incomplete.

Consuming fat from long-ago meals, shades
perfect their hibernation until hunger
nudges the sleeper out. At times, in face-like
ripples of a swollen moon, or mirrored
behind the rows of overhandled fruit
where I shop, I acknowledge her form.
Reaching out for purple plums my hand brushes
hers. Our tired and solitary eyes meet,
then I turn, buy another book, and go on back.

Matchmaking

Stephany Brown

The adjustor wrote my mother a letter. Dear Mrs. Delaney, the adjustor wrote, I used to know your daughter. Don't tell me any more, I said to my mother, don't tell me any more.

I had no idea which one of my bandana-wearing boyfriends could have turned into an adjustor, whatever an adjustor is, but there was no curiosity anywhere inside of me about any of it. I just wanted to feed and dress my girls and myself, get them to school and me to work, make a few Play-Doh sculptures after dinner, read a few Babar books, brush and floss my teeth, and get into bed. Alone. If I had heard then that all the men had gone, gone to soldiers or to flowers or whatever, that would have been just fine with me.

I knew that my mother would copy that letter and put it in the mail to me and that I would throw it in the trash can without looking at it. I knew that I'd be on the lookout for short-haired men in grey suits coming up my walk, just in case she'd given the adjustor my address. I wouldn't open the door, I said. I wouldn't look at the face.

My mother has these parties. Dogwood blossoms in pink vases on highly polished tables. Silver trays covered in lettuce and then arty little canapés. She swishes around in blue silk or green, her silver hair perfect. Her friends are there, mostly married couples but a few courting couples, widowers courting widows, like Mr. Larson and my mother. And there's always a divorced or never married son of one of the friends. A lawyer or architect or stockbroker. Once even a carpenter. There for me, of course. But I no longer attend my mother's parties.

I went home with one of those men once. To my house. He drove the baby-sitter home. He came back. I had sobered up a little by then and didn't want him to be there. I knew there'd be a scene. I sliced some cake, I made some tea. I put on a record. I remember looking for something that might tame a libido. I chose a brisk violin concerto, something that made me hold my head erect and sit straight in my chair. Strings. Lots of strings. Something to pay bills by or arrange flowers. But it was too late for Bob; Bob was his name. He wanted to dance. I said, no, I don't know how to dance to Mozart. I said, how about a movie tomorrow night, there's an old Truffaut at the Biograph. But it was too late for Bob. You know how men are. Bob's khaki pants came off, my stockings got ripped. The children were sleeping. I didn't scream. Bob had his way with me. Bob went home. I hate Bob.

My mother called the next day, all cheerful, all expectant. I told her not to get her hopes up, that Bob and I don't really have that much in common, but that sure, we might have dinner together sometime. I was on the portable phone, and as we talked I walked to my closet and picked my party clothes up off the floor and carried them into the kitchen where I buried them, deep in the garbage. We kept talking, my mother and I, about the canapés and how nice the silver had looked. We talked about Mr. and Mrs. Foster, wintering in Florida really suits them. Mrs. McNaughton had had several manhattans. We shouldn't have let her drive even those few blocks home, should we have. I said I had to hang up. Sophie and Isabel had to get ready for a party.

Bob wasn't the carpenter. I don't remember what he did by day. Securities, maybe, or the stock exchange. A dream son-in-law for my mother. He'd buy me a grey Audi and take me on airplane vacations. The girls would have violins and lessons on Thursdays. We'd have health insurance and all new clothes. Fluoride treatments. Bob. Go back to hell, Bob.

Isabel and Sophie covered themselves in lace and bows and carried their presents up the walk to Adam's house. A panther was delivering balloons at the same time. I had two hours alone. I wanted to go to a decontamination chamber. I felt like Meryl Streep in *Silkwood*. I wanted my insides scrubbed with Brillo pads. I wanted to throw up, again and again.

I drove to the hospital and sat in the parking lot. I pictured sitting in a clean, white room and talking to a doctor. He would be taking notes, avoiding my face. He would tell the nurse to get the rape kit. He would comb my pubic hair, swab my insides, smear stuff on slides. The police would come. A female officer. Dark blue uniform. Shiny gold badge. I would tell her Bob's last name. I pictured meeting Bob in the courtroom. I saw his smirk. I heard the judge's gavel hit wood. Case dismissed? Guilty? Innocent? What did it matter? I drove away.

I drove to my mother's house and sat on her lawn. Her car was gone, but that was OK. I had nothing to tell her. She'd see my unwashed hair, the dark half-moons under my eyes, and ask if I was OK. Maybe she'd notice my bitten fingernails. The night before, at the party, they'd been perfect ovals, perfect raspberry glacé ovals.

Shiny cars passed. Hedge trimmers buzzed. Lilacs bloomed. Bright green grasshoppers hopped. Mr. Larson, from next door, came over in his white shoes and Old Spice. He had a key in his hand attached to a ring I'd made at camp. Gimp. I'd braided it with gimp. The key was to my mother's back door. The Larsons had always had the key, even before Mrs. Larson died, even before Mr. Larson started courting my mother. Here, honey, Mr. Larson said, go on inside. You don't want to sit out here on the wet ground. My throat closed when he called me honey, and then I started to cry. He didn't know what to do. I covered my face with my hands. I didn't want anyone to ever treat me kindly again.

I took the key and headed for the backyard. I called out to Mr. Larson not to worry, that I was fine. I just needed to borrow my mother's soufflé dish.

The kitchen counters gleamed with silver from the party: fluted compote dishes, candelabra, flatware carefully dried and laid in rows. My mother likes rows. She rolls her underpants and lays them in rows in her sacheted pink-lined top drawer. Her snapdragons grow in a perfect row. If a seed strays and a plant comes up, she plucks it out, she won't even wait for it to flower. And in the afternoon, after she makes her first drink, she puts everything away, the tonic, the gin, the ice. She wipes the counter. As if she won't return to make a second drink, a third, a fourth. I opened a drawer. The dish towels were rolled up and placed in a row. I slammed the drawer shut.

My mother's party wasn't the first time I'd seen Bob. He and his dad and my father and Marie, my athletic sister, used to play tennis together sometimes. He'd come to the door to pick up my dad and Marie, or they'd stop by after their games for lemonade. Bob was a few years younger than I, I didn't pay him too much attention. We were all invited to his wedding, though. I didn't attend, but I was with my mother when she chose the gift. We checked the Bridal Registry. His bride wanted silver and china and crystal. We chose a silver pie server and a slotted spoon and a pair of tongs for sugar cubes. That's what she wanted, it was all checked off on the form. Rambling Rose was the name of their pattern. Towle? Gorham?

"Rambling Rose" was one of the songs Mr. Larson played at the party. Mom always asks Mr. Larson to help with the music. Nat King Cole. I don't know where Bob and I were as Nat belted it out. Standing by the potted palm talking about expressionism in painting? Walking down the long hallway, my mother's photo gallery, looking at pictures of me and my sisters at different stages of our lives? Or putting on our coats, being kissed good-bye by all those red lips, heading out the door?

We had stopped at a picture of me and my five sisters. I don't know what was on the stereo. The picture shows us on a boat, somewhere out in the Chesapeake Bay, sailboats off in the hazy distance. It had been our father's boat, and we had just thrown his ashes over the side. My mother had taken the picture. I was telling Bob about that day and about what had happened to the ashes when they hit the air. I was trying to replay the conversation my sisters and my mother and I had had. Bob just kept looking at the pictures of us and asking questions about our ages, our education, our jobs, how many children we had, as if he were deciding which one of us to hire. He seemed most interested in Janie. Her looks are the most dramatic. Obsidian hair, a boyfriend had once written in a poem, sea green eyes. She always got to play Snow White when we were small. Her body is willowy and her lips are like Kim Basinger's. Poutier lips in the picture than usual; she'd been crying. Bob didn't care about her tears. How high up is she in the organization? he'd wanted to know about her job at CBS. When was she at Skidmore? Does she play racquetball? I was on my third or fourth glass of wine by then. I didn't mind the questions.

At some point Mr. Larson put on Glen Miller. "In the Mood" maybe. He didn't know how to jitterbug, Bob said with disdain when I asked him. Didn't matter to me. Mr. Cunningham, my parents' friend and dentist, was always good for a dance. My mother got a little tight-lipped when I danced with the old men, but I thought it made them happy. I never minded making people happy. And we never knocked the figurines off the end tables. Just relax, Mother.

My mother always wants everything to look right. It doesn't look right for a thirty-five-year-old to dance with a sixty-five-year-old. It doesn't look right for a bottle of gin to stand exposed on a patio table. It doesn't look right for a woman to live alone with her two daughters. So it was a shock to step into her living room the day after her party and see the records all askew. I set about putting them in order, in alphabetical order. My mother came in the front door, her arms loaded with dry cleaning and groceries. Oh, honey, are you sick? she said, when she'd taken a good look. My throat closed, and I turned to the record albums. Doesn't it annoy you, I said, that Mr. Larson leaves these things in such a mess after your parties? I mean, he could at least put the records back in their sleeves. Doesn't he know they get ruined when he just stacks vinyl against vinyl? And the old records, the ones that are really valuable, take the worst beating. What are they made of, anyway? They're so brittle. Look at this old Artie Shaw. Scratched to death. And he's so fastidious about his stupid yard.

She apologized, as if it were my living room that had been left untidy. She said she didn't really know what the old records were made of, some kind of early vinyl, she supposed. Had I gotten enough sleep? she wanted to know.

Oh, sure, I said, and looked at my watch. Gotta go, I said, Sophie and Isabel's party ends at four. She wondered if we shouldn't all go out to dinner, her treat. No, thanks, I said, scared to give her the time to mention Bob again. Then how about ordering a pizza and bringing the girls by? I could go home and take a nap, she said, she could tell I needed one. Thanks, Mom, I said, maybe tomorrow night. I knew I didn't want to be alone.

I made it to Adam's house OK and hugged the girls hard. When I kissed Sophie's cheek I got a taste of icing—confectioner's sugar and Crisco. I made small talk with the other mothers, I congratulated the birthday boy. I rushed the girls to the car.

As we drove home I tried not to think about it, tried to pay attention to the pin-the-tail-on-the-dinosaur story and the fun of duck, duck, goose. But I kept seeing pieces of the night before, the Rolex on Bob's wrist as he handed me my first drink, the Rolex again before he pinned down my arms. He actually looked at it as if everything were happening on a schedule. I saw the white teeth in the smile when I said, sure, he could follow me home. And I saw those same white teeth, bared, furious, later, when I spit in his face. I saw the red and yellow suns on his hand-painted canvas tie, our conversation opener. Did you paint it yourself? I'd wanted to know. It was a gift, he'd said. A friend to artists, I remember thinking. A sensitive man.

The phone was ringing when we got home. Isabel ran for it. She loved to answer the phone. I screamed at her, loud and mean. Don't you dare go near that phone, I said, as if it were in flames. She turned to me, stunned. Why, Mommy? Because. Because it might be somebody bad. What a terrifying thing to tell a child. But I didn't recant, didn't fold her into my arms. Go change out of your party dresses, I said. And do it right away. My voice was cruel. Sophie started to cry. And none of that, I said.

I don't know who I thought was on the phone. Certainly not Bob. Bob wanting to bring pizza over? Bob wanting me to pack a picnic basket for a Sunday sail? Bob wanting to run out and catch *Jules and Jim* at the Biograph?

Mommy, can we have macaroni and cheese for dinner? It was Isabel, Isabel trying to make peace, Isabel giving me a chance, generous, wise Isabel. Sure, honey, if you'll help me make it.

After dinner there was a bath, a long one with foam that squirts out of a can and curls like fat spaghetti. I stared at my face in the mirror as Isabel and Sophie squirted and squealed. Did I look like a whore? I asked myself. A little mascara had smeared. Did I look like a mother? My black hair hung down like a veil, and I could see a few strands of white. I looked at my neck, my arms. I saw no scars. Maybe the beginnings of finger bruises. No big deal.

We washed hair. We dried hair. We sprinkled powder. We jumped on the bed. My bed. I opened the window. There were dead bees on the sill. Five dead bees. Yellow jackets.

His car pulled up, his sleek red car. He got out. I stepped behind the curtain, a woman in a movie. Stop jumping. Lie down on the bed. My voice was cruel again. I looked through the lace, at his madras shirt, his deck shoes, at the white package he held in his hand. It looked like a roast. Deer meat from his last hunting trip? I remembered the contempt in his voice at the party when he spoke of his ex-wife: she'd disapproved of hunting. Could he really have been bringing me a venison roast as a peace offering? Did he want me to stick it in the oven? Put some potatoes on to boil, throw together a salad? We could put the girls to bed, put linen and silver on the table, light the candles. Paganini on the stereo. He could hold my bitten hand.

Don't move, I said to the girls. I closed the bedroom door and walked downstairs. He was still at the door. I could smell him.

I have a gun, Bob, I said. Get away from my door, or I'll blow your brains out.

I didn't look out the window. He didn't run to his car, but he didn't linger either. The red door slammed shut. The engine shrieked, and then Bob was gone. He never came back, and that was a long time ago.

Now the only one I've got to worry about is the adjustor. The damned adjustor who wrote my mother a letter. Dear Mrs. Delaney, the adjustor wrote, I used to know your daughter. Don't tell me any more, I said to my mother, don't tell me any more.

Response to a Reading

Michele Wolf

For Li-Young Lee

In two of your poems you called that central
Passage of womanhood a wound,
Instead of a curtain guarding a silken
Trail of sighs. How many men,
Upon regarding such beauty, helplessly
Touching it, recklessly needing
To enter its warmth again and again,
Have assumed it embodies their own ache
Of absence, the personal
Gash that has punished their lives.
So endowed of anatomy, any woman
Who has been loved
Knows that her tenderest blush
Of tissue is a luxe burden of have.
Although it bleeds, this is only to cleanse,
To prepare yet another nesting for love.
It is not a wound, friend.
It is a home for you.
It is a way into the world.

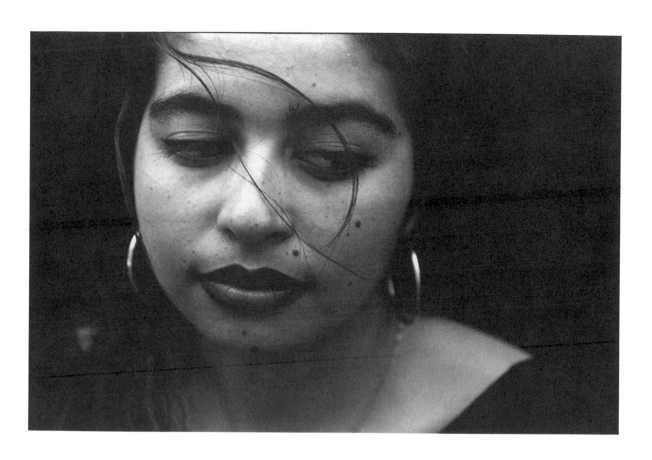

What I Know from Noses

Anndee Hochman

From the time I was eight years old, I understood that noses, even if they were not broken, could be mended.

My aunt had had a nose job, and she wasn't shy about it. I sat next to her on the couch while we paged through old photo albums. "There I am with my old nose," she sometimes said, as if the old nose were a childhood friend who had moved away.

I never asked my aunt why she had her nose fixed. The question seemed too obvious. The old one was too big and too bumpy. Who would pick a bumpy nose, a Jewish nose, if she had the choice? My aunt's new nose looked normal—not too wide or too thin, not too flared at the nostrils or uneven at the bridge. Not a nose anyone would look at twice in a crowded elevator. Which was, I guessed, the idea.

My aunt seemed happy with her new nose. When she smiled, her whole face thrilled—her teeth gleamed and her cheekbones nudged upward, and her nose did not do anything at all. Everyone in the family said she was very photogenic. I thought she was beautiful.

I am in high school, sitting in music class. The wooden chair prods hard against my back; tears burn my eyes. I am fifteen. At just under five feet, I've grown as tall as I'm going to get, and my body has changed. In the sixth grade, my straight dark hair crinkled first into waves, then wiry, unruly kinks. I'm no longer underweight. And my nose, true to family form, has developed a bump.

I look at photographs from before I grew, before my face turned traitor, and I want to cry. I rub my finger down the length of my nose. It feels huge where the bone rises. I think it is growing. At home, with the bathroom door locked, I turn sideways in front of the mirror and hold one hand over my nose, imagining how much better I'd look if it fell straight and smooth from bridge to tip.

On buses, in department stores, at the movies, I see noses attached to people. I judge the noses—too big, too snubbed, better than mine, worse than mine. I hardly see any that are worse than mine.

I am determined not to cry in music class. But Bob Fitzsimmons has just called me "suicide slope." Not for the first time. Across the room, he is snickering about my nose, his shoulders twitching as he whispers to the boy sitting next to him. Bob Fitzsimmons has too many freckles, he wears ugly clothes, and I hate him. I hate my nose.

After dinner that night, I sob to my mother. Everyone thinks I'm ugly, I tell her. I want a new nose. I want this one fixed. She hugs me tightly. OK, she says, OK. We'll go see some doctors.

I started my junior year in high school with crisp looseleaf binders, several medium-point black Bic pens, and a new nose. The operation wasn't so bad. At one point I started to surface out of the anesthesia and felt someone tapping in the middle of my face. It didn't hurt; it just felt annoying, like a headache you wish would go away.

For a week, I wore a bandage and didn't leave the house; for the rest of the summer, I had to be careful not to let my nose get sunburned. In August my father took a picture of me standing on our front walk. I had let my hair grow long since school let out; I wore a wide-brimmed straw hat and a white sundress. I angled my head at the camera, letting my nose show, and smiled widely. It was the first photograph of myself I remember liking.

Back at school, my life was much the same as the year before. I got A's in my classes, wrote for the newspaper, woke up at 6:15 every morning so I could spend forty-five minutes blow-drying the curls out of my hair. But inside myself, I felt changed.

My boyfriend told me, in cramped printing on a sheepishly sweet card, that he thought I was pretty. I believed him. When I acted in school plays, I didn't hesitate to turn my profile to the audience. And on buses, eventually, I stopped noticing the noses first.

More than a decade later, I'm still just barely five feet tall and weigh the same as I did at fifteen. In college I quit wrestling my hair straight; now I wash it and let it dry in random curls. I rarely use makeup. In the summer, I shave my legs from the knees down. "My concession to polite society," I tell my mother.

Sometimes I stand in line at Safeway, turning the glossy pages of women's magazines. Hair dyes, depilatories, plastic surgeries, polymer fingernails, page after page of creams and blushes and eyeliners and lip glosses, page after page of implicit promises: Use this and you'll be beautiful, slender, deliriously happy. These women don't look like me; they don't look like anyone I've ever met. I stuff the magazines back in their racks and pay for my tofu, my spinach, my mineral water. I feel pleased that I'm not buying nail polish.

As a matter of principle, I declare I will never dye grey out of my hair, wear blue contact lenses on my brown eyes, or buy clothes that feel terrible just because they're in style. I tell myself that wearing one's natural face out in the world is not only an honest act, but a political one.

And for all these fourteen years I have carried a secret glitch in my principles, a bump as big as an old nose.

Unlike my aunt, I never talked about my nose job once I left high school. Not even my lovers knew. If friends came to visit at my parents' house, I made sure they saw only baby pictures with my cute snub of a nose, not the telltale "before" photos of adolescence.

It wasn't the nose itself that bothered me so much as the raw spot in my consciousness. I didn't want to remember a time of cringing at nose jokes and hiding my profile from my father's camera. I didn't want to recall how I stung with embarrassment and shame and the desperate hunger to look "right."

As I grew older, questions and arguments haunted my decision. Who says a bumpy nose is bad? Who cares what people think? Why is it mostly Jewish girls who get their noses fixed, Jewish noses that poke across the boundaries of what is considered beautiful? If you change a part of your physical self permanently, what happens to the intangible parts; does your psyche also shift to fit the new shape?

Sometimes, in the bathroom with the door locked, I looked in the mirror and cupped my hand against my nose, making a space where the bump used to be. I wondered then what I had lost when I asked the surgeon to scrape my bone down to smooth—and how I could get it back.

In the last few years, I have begun to tell friends about my nose. The whole story comes back to me vividly: the burn I felt at fifteen, wanting so badly to be pretty. The relief afterward, then all the years of embarrassed, guilty silence. And this realization: that when I stopped seeing noses everywhere I turned, my vision gained room for other things—my whole self, people around me, the desires that webbed us together.

Maybe I would have shed that self-consciousness anyway, slipped gradually out of it and into adulthood. Maybe if I hadn't had a nose job, I would be the same person I am now, just with a rougher profile. I don't believe that chromosomes drive destiny. But I do know that removing the bump on my nose somehow helped me to see past it.

If I ever have a daughter, and her nose takes after mine, and it makes her miserable, I'm not sure what I will tell her. Maybe I'll discuss sexist codes of attractiveness and tell her she's gorgeous just as she is. Maybe I'll hold her tightly and say, OK, let's go talk to some doctors.

I would want my daughter to know this: On the subject of women and beauty, it is the rules, not our bodies, that need repair. But even as I talk, I will remember myself at fifteen—how much, how fervently I wanted and deserved to feel fixed.

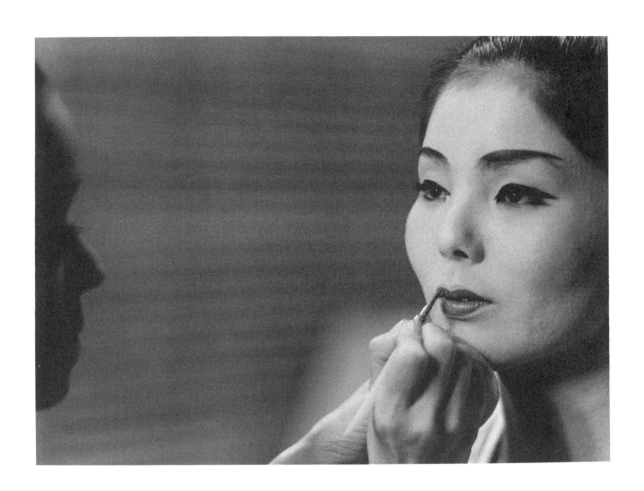

The Makeup Poem

Jan Epton Seale

There is a garden in her face
—Thomas Campion

Yes, it is
frivolous
expensive
time-consuming
artificial
dangerous
and unworthy.

Yes, it mimes
the posterior
sexual colorations
of the adult
male mandrill.

Yes, the number
of products
pawned off
on women,
with "rev-"
"-some"
and "-ique"
in their names
is indeed
scandalous.

No, a woman's face
can't need
toner, blusher,
liner, smudger,
powder, cover,
enhancer—

plus base,
lotion, stick,
and rouge
all at once.

And yes, I shall wear it.
For: The names are beautiful.
This is closet art.
Men without are not better
than women with.
Nature loves a color display.
Clowns and mimes are magic.

Ode to Grey Hair

Alisa Wolf

"It's only one grey hair," my mother said. She glanced at me over her shoulder, already on her way back to the bedroom where she'd been ironing shirts in front of the afternoon movie.

I stared into the bathroom mirror and separated the glittering hair from its darker sisters. "You!" I said. "You made me old before my time, before I could leave my mother's house, graduate high school, make love." I raked my scalp for more grey, sifted through the brown strands I'd been growing for seventeen years, imagining they made me luscious.

My mother passed by with an empty laundry basket on her hip. "Don't pull it out," she said. "It'll only grow back double."

While she watched, I yanked it out by the root.

"If you don't like it, Margery, you can dye it. It's not the end of the world."

"Easy for you to say, Mom." She must have been twenty-nine when I came home from third grade and found her in bed, the door to her room half ajar, her head buried so deeply under blankets that all but the ends of her brown curls stayed hidden. My father drove up early from the office and passed in and out of their bedroom all afternoon. I hung around the hallway, hearing my mother's weeping and his soft voice reassuring. He made spaghetti for dinner, but even that didn't draw her out. I didn't see her again until the next afternoon, when I came home from school and found her at the kitchen table with the phone cradled between shoulder and chin, laughing into the receiver, her hair glazed with unfamiliar cherry highlights.

"You freaked out when you went grey." I stood in the doorway of her bedroom almost ten years later, one hand on the doorknob, the other on my hip, ready to defend my truth. But she didn't challenge me. Instead, she fussed so long with one of my father's blue shirts, I started to lose confidence.

"Leave your mother alone," she finally said, hanging the shirt up and turning back to the set. "I'm trying to watch this movie."

She was right about the grey. It returned. It brought its cousins from overseas, sold my follicles to its friends, married, had babies. Meanwhile I went to college, studied astronomy and anatomy, biology and Bettelheim, tried to settle on a major, and avoided my reflection in bathroom mirrors. By the time I'd earned a liberal arts degree, property values on my scalp had plummeted. There goes the neighborhood, I thought, as the grey spread out of control. I rallied my dark hairs, begging them: Hold fast! Hang onto your roots.

At Thanksgiving dinner during my twenty-fifth year, my grey hair attracted Aunt Helen's gaze. "You know," she said, "your Nana is as dark-haired as she was at your age."

Nana's head was bent over a plate of pumpkin pie. She wore her black locks, as always, oiled with VO5 and coiled into a bun. She looked up from her plate, from my aunt to me. "What did you say?"

Aunt Helen touched her dark curls. "I must have inherited your genes, Ma!"

Then whose evil gene snuck into my pool? Does grey hair blow like seeds in the wind, take root in scalps fertilized with bad living, late nights, skipped breakfasts? My mother tipped back her chair and sucked on a toothpick from the olive tray. She didn't look too thrilled. Did she think I blamed her? Did I worry too much about what she thought? Would I be going grey now had I got the hang of the carefree girls, their blond pony-tails flung over their boyfriends' school jackets? Would I be less grey now had I taken a job rather than sweating out a dissertation? Did I study too hard, take myself too seriously, spend too little time on the important things?

On my way home Sunday afternoon, I stopped at the mall near the apartment I shared with my lover, Kate. We lived in East Cambridge, an old immigrant neighborhood crammed full with wooden houses divided into units of two, three, four, and more. Every now and then one caught fire, damaging a whole block in minutes. We had two fresh fish stores—one Portuguese, one Italian—down on Cambridge Street, and a place that smelled of sawdust and advertised "Fresh Killed Chickens" over its door. The corner stores still sold coffee and donuts, newspapers, and canned goods, their old wooden shelves dusty and sparsely stocked. But for anything major, you had to go to the mall.

My mother told me she didn't know what color her hair would be if she let the dye grow out. Once you start dying your hair, she warned, you had to touch up the roots regularly, and keep it up. OK, I told myself, and I followed the stink of hair care products down the drugstore aisles until I found, between the eye shadows and the shampoos, the boxes featuring female faces buoyed by hair. Each brand was arranged on a color spectrum from blond to black, with every variation in between: reds and browns, ash colors and warm. They were lined up Warhol-like, the same face over and over again on the shelf. I chose the face with the kindest eyes and the hair color closest to my own dark brown, and bought a supply of low-commitment shampoo-in dye to last me a year.

I unloaded the plastic drugstore bag and lined up my brown-eyed Rapunzels under the bathroom sink. Hair swept over each right eye, one luscious wave after another. I felt rich. I attacked my head that night, while Kate drove back from her family celebration three states away. I sudsed in the dye, arranged my hair in the plastic cap provided, and set the timer on the stove.

If only Kate had been fifteen minutes later. As it was, she caught me dripping in the hallway, a white towel around my neck ringed with brown.

"Don't hug me. I'll stain you."

"What? Margie, what are you doing?"

"Dying my hair." I crossed my arms over my terry cloth robe.

Kate took a step closer and peered at my head.

"Don't come any closer. How was your trip?"

"You look like a mad surgeon or something. Why are you doing that?"

I'd begun to laugh, a silent, heaving laugh, and talking made it harder to keep it in control. "My aunt," I started, "she said I had more grey hair than my Nana." I took a deep breath.

"Your aunt? So what?"

"I'll tell you later." I held my stomach and tried to breathe deeply. The timer went off. "I gotta go," I warbled. "I'll get too dark."

"You'd better," Kate said. "There's brown stuff dripping down your neck. Won't it come out when you go swimming?"

I shook my head, the laugh in my gut clenched like a sob, and fled to the bathroom where I rinsed in the shower. I emerged that night with hair as dark and natural looking as the package had promised.

It wasn't until Monday morning, after my first cup of coffee, that I realized just how dramatic the change really was. In the sunlight shining through the window over the sink, my hair glowed with a hard, metallic shine, a red sheen that spread uniformly over the top of my head.

There was no way it wouldn't be noticed.

"So you dyed your hair!" my mother said. "And that was going to be my Chanukah present to you."

She handed me an envelope which held a card and a gift certificate for Le Salon des Belles. "Oh, well. You can still use it. See how it feels to be done by a pro. Maybe Philip can help you find the right color."

"What's wrong with the color?"

"Now don't get all excited, Margery."

"It's too dark, isn't it?"

"The color's fine."

I glanced again at the gift certificate. "You really went all out."

"Listen, Margery. Use it for whatever you want. A new cut, a manicure, a rinse, anything you like. I want you to feel good about yourself."

"Something's different about you," was the neutral comment I mostly heard.

When I answered, "I dyed my hair," friends were delighted.

"You look much better," they said. "Your face is much too young for grey hair."

My Aunt Helen was especially pleased. "Believe me," she said, "it will help you find a man."

One night that week, I found myself watching a grey-haired PBS anchorwoman. "Imagine," I told Kate, "letting your hair grey in front of the cameras like that."

"It looks pretty."

The woman was forty, tops, and her hair gleamed—long, sleek, and white. I couldn't take my eyes off her.

Now, on the subway, I seek the grey women, a silver brigade with white halos and fluffy spots of brown, fading like tans in winter. Downtown, I watch long grey hair flow down the back of black coats. Older women cross my path, their hair bright white, blazing. I look for greying temples, steel grey cut short, silver streaks, and soft white curls. On TV I search for the grey celebrities: Bea Arthur, Barbara Bush, the PBS anchorwoman. My list grows long.

Still, at Le Salon des Belles, Philip wants to hide my grey with cellophane rinse or eggplant wash. He tempts me with colors from sun-white blond to blue-black, tells me I'm too young to put up with grey hair, and frankly, it's compromising my looks. His palette, locks of synthetic fibers dipped down the spectrum, mimics the boxes in the drugstore. I can almost taste the tang of orange-red, the mintiness of paper-bag brown, the smooth, creamy comfort of dark chocolate.

"Someday, maybe," I tell him. I haven't ruled it out.

After my haircut, I confronted my grey hair again in the bathroom mirror. There it was, its presence harder than ever to ignore.

I looked under the sink, and the woman with the warm brown flounce smiled out at me. I picked out a box, turned it over. *Gentle, easy, controllable, fast,* the back panel read in bold letters, neatly arranged.

You, grey hair, a wild weed, a witch's prerogative. You, my enemy, my nemesis, my harbinger. "You," I said, patting you down. "What do you promise?"

"Nothing," you whispered, your voice hoarse with old age or older. "Nothing."

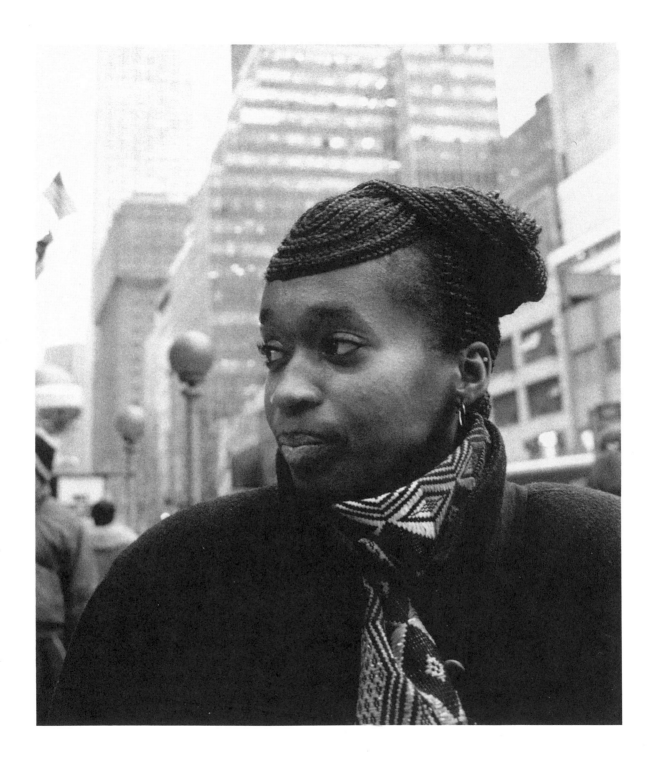

Shell Life

Shirley Vogler Meister

This is my imperfect shell: hold it
to your heart to hear the hidden hymns
of me as Sheena, harmonizing
in the jungle heat with more beastly
sounds—or me as Salome, jangling
with jewels midst gossamery veils
of seduction—or Ginger Rogers,
with agile legs deftly tapping out
tunes of tender rhythm and romance—
or sturdy Pioneer, steadily
trudging to the drumbeats of control—
or Holy Woman, whose chants confirm
unchangeable links to life and love—
or Mother, crooning sweet lullabies
to those who will grow into their own
imperfect shells, hoping for others
to hold them against listening hearts.

La Maja Desnuda

Anne M. Candelaria

Do not mistake my plainness
for lack of passion.
I look at Southern women
sway and display
their sexuality
And want to make myself over
Put on false eyelashes
and long fingernails
Bleach my hair
pluck a thin line of eyebrow
Leave my cleavage exposed
But I feel silly doing this
Like dressing up
in costume.
Come feel my thighs
so dimpled and lush,
Notice my breasts
pointed classically outward,
My cheeks rosy with health,
My eyes brown with intelligence.
Am I not more
like Goya's women
than those practiced sirens?
Grab my unpainted hand,
kiss my modestly
rouged mouth
Press me to you.
You will find fire there,
Stoked by pages of poetry,
literary lunges, much praying.

Living the Green Life
Maril Crabtree

Shocking to see these bearded
calves where ice-blank smoothness
met my eyes before. Not since

age twelve were my legs thus
adorned with dark, thick hair so
long it curls upon itself. Why

grow hair now? My friends ask.
It has something to do with
tenderness, I say. These

legs deserve a rest after
almost forty years of
being daily scraped, sometimes

hastily, brutally, almost
always thoughtlessly, into
someone else's idea of

beauty. My neighbor concludes
the same about his lawn: no more
harsh chemicals, grass mowed to

within an inch of its roots.
Let it grow, let it luxuriate
au naturel. My legs, his lawn:

we are about reforestation,
he and I, reclaiming the wild, preserving the native state of things.

The Spearthrower

Lillian Morrison

She walks alone
to the edge of the park
and throws into
the bullying dark
her javelin
of light,
her singing sign
her signed song
that the runner may run
far and long
her quick laps
on the curving track,
that the sprinter surge
and the hurdler leap,
that the vaulter soar,
clear the highest bar,
and the discus fly
as the great crowds cry
to their heroines
Come on!

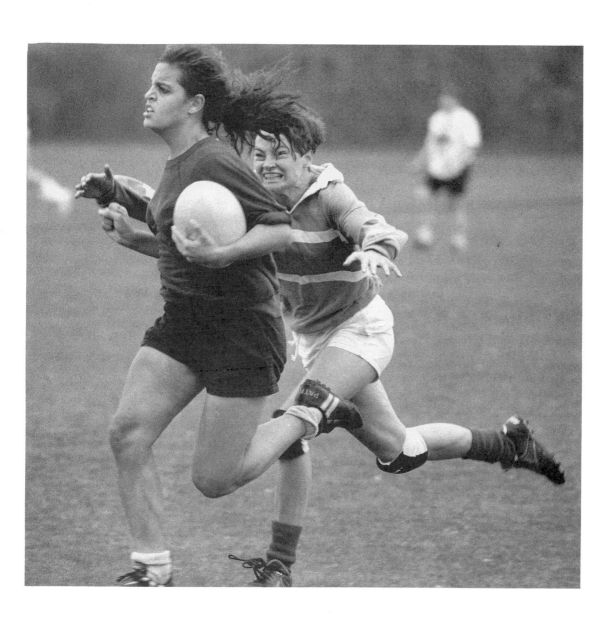

The Marathon

Marnie Mueller

Strategy

I will start
when the gun goes off.
I will run
for five miles.
Feeling good,
I will run
to the tenth mile.
At the tenth
I will say,
"Only three more
to halfway."

At the halfway mark
I will know
fifteen is in reach.
At fifteen miles
I will say,
"You've run twenty before,
keep going."
At twenty
I will say,
"Run home."

The Race

We start
when the gun goes off.
We climb the Verrazano Narrows
five thousand strong
running toward the metropolis

anchored in the water.
We ride the crest.
At one mile
a thousand breaths exhale
propel us downhill
to the second.
Overhead
helicopters
their chatter superfluous
to pounding feet
and hopes
their noise finally
submerged
in embracing cheers
of family, friends, and strangers
awaiting us
on that first shore.

Mile two.

At mile three
she joins me, a woman
of my same height, weight, and age.
Five feet five and one half
one hundred and twenty pounds
thirty-five years old.
"Hello, I'm Caryl.
Do I know you?"
"Yes, I'm Marnie.
I met you at a meeting
of the track club."
We laugh at our presumptuousness.

"Is this your first?"
"Yes, yours too?"
"Yes."

We run together
matching strides.
We hold ourselves back
computing times at each mile
afraid of speeding up
straining to leap forward.
She, the more sensible,
recalls this is the time of temptation.
I, the more reckless,
resent her moderation.
"I must remember," she says,
"If I go too fast now, I won't have it
when I need it."
I'm the stronger, I think,
I will pick up my speed, in time,
and shake her.

Mile six.

A long straightaway
unrolls to the Manhattan skyline.
Spots of color bobble for miles ahead.
Two blocks away the spots take shape
round, square, triangular, oblong.
Closer still, they become
tall, fat, short, skinny.
Around me, they begin
to have ages, faces, breasts, and buttocks.

We are two orange-and-blue spots.
She, light skinned and blond.
I, brown and brown.
"Yeah for the ladies."
"Hooray for F180 and F210."
"Keep it up girls."
Black children line the way
extending tan palms to be touched
by the runners
by us.

Mile ten.

Brooklyn is endless
miles are longer in Brooklyn
Hasidic Jews stop time in Brooklyn.
They crowd together on corners as we pass
chortling over our physicality.

Do they know I'm menstruating, I wonder?
Would they blanch in horror at the knowledge,
shrinking from my presence
to huddle in a clot backward up stairs
to safe houses of learning?
Far from Jewish women like myself,
the ultimate betrayers
whose strong legs and backs
transport minds as ancient
as their own.

Mile twelve.

At last,
"Thirteen point one miles
your time is two hours and two minutes
you have reached the halfway point,"
at the summit of the Pulaski bridge,
Manhattan towers overhead
reminding me of home.
It's quiet on the bridge
and white with sunlight.
My colleague runs beside me
straight and tall.
"You look good," I say.
She smiles.
"I like the silence," I say.
She nods.

Down into Queens
into the arms of
screaming mobs.
Just in time
a bagpipe band lifts the spirits.

Then there appears on the corner of a commercial street
amidst beer-drinking howling bulbous men, a woman,
dressed in frayed full-sleeved black coat, waving a homemade
flag of pink satin panties trimmed in antique lace.

From all around
come hoots
and laughter
of male runners,
my comrades of the hour.

I resist my rage
but our community is broken.

Mile fifteen.

We approach the 59th Street bridge
the one they've warned of
and carpeted in electric blue
to save our feet.
We mount it from the side.

Cars honk harshly traveling against us.
The city's granite walls now could crush us.
The water is dangerously far below.
Where is the rug that's supposed to help us?
Where is the Allen Carpet rug?

And then, softly, we step softly
treacherously softly
onto
the mile
of miracle fibers
leading to Manhattan.

It's too narrow! Too narrow to run abreast!
I take the lead. Is she with me? I glance behind. Yes.
"Look, Marnie, our shadows, on the water, how beautiful."
I can't look down.

Runners ahead begin to slow. I must risk the grating or
curtail our progress. I must leave the carpet. I must
move suspended over space far above our gallant shadows.

I meet the challenge. I move out. Can she keep up?
Would she prefer the rest? I turn back to look as she
too steps out of line picking up her pace.

Mile sixteen.

We plunge
into Manhattan
trace a wide arch on the asphalt surface.
The sun
craning around buildings
rejoices
the streets echo with accolades
for warriors entering the city
succulent oranges
sweet chocolate
proffered by East Side dowagers
savagely consumed
by us
the victors.

We live dreams
on First Avenue
We feed dreams
on First Avenue
We kill dreams
on First Avenue
as
in conference
she
and I
recall our own

mortality
and
slow
our pace.
In that
instant
it
becomes
our race.

Mile seventeen.

In El Barrio
ellos gritan
"Gringa, Gringa"
reminding me
of the distance
I have traveled
today
soy una extranjera
aqui
where ten years before
fuí
amiga.
Ahora
I help myself
Ayuda
Ayuda
Socorro
Now the white women struggle
in the street.
Por qué?

Nineteen.

To leave home before arriving
To be finished before completing
We enter the Bronx
We begin the twentieth mile
Fuzzy Wuzzy was a bear
Fuzzy Wuzzy had no hair
fuzzy wuzzy is my head
my legs are made of lead
I cannot think ahead
I want to go to bed
I want to walk
not run
bask in October sun
be carefree and light
and silly and free
and not take myself so
seriously.

London Bridge is falling down falling down falling down
London Bridge is falling down,
my fair lady
We are now walking up walking up walking up,
We are now walking up,
the Willis Avenue
Bridge
out of Manhattan
into the Bronx
away from the goal
go on without me
Why won't she leave?

I'm holding her back.
STUUPIID friend
ly
woman
RUUUNNNN.
"I'm staying with you," she insists.
She walks beside me.
I can't shake her now.

Oh, Mama, how much further to go?
Oh, Mama, my feet are so cold.
Oh, Mama, carry me home.
Oh, Mama, sing me a song.

Oh! Susanna
Sing Mama, please Mama, help me along.
Oh, don't you cry for me
I come from Alabama with a banjo on my knee.
"I can't go on."
"I think you can."
"My legs won't move."
"We've come this far."
"I know. You're right. I have to try."
Oh! Susanna

then
one   leg   begins   to power   the body
the   other   follows suit
the first holds firm
and we're off again
in quest of our full term.

Oh, don't you cry for me
I've come from Alabama with a banjo on my knee.

Returning to Manhattan,
we carry our tiredness
through Harlem streets
"Looking good girl"
"Do it for me"
me
me
me
"Put it there girl"
girl
girl
girl
on my sandpaper palm
pull
pull
pull
me along
long
long
long
not long to go
go
go
girl
girl
do it for me

Catch a lizard by the tail and you're left
holding the tail.

Amputate a portion of a leaf, take a special photograph
and you capture its essence.
Try to fall off a bike once you've learned to ride
and you'll find you can't.

Central Park.
Scarlet maples against October sky
golden ginkgo fans scatter into green.
Light surrounds us.
The sun crusts sweat to salt
on the surface of our skin.

Happy faces dart out in our path, people jump up and down
around us our names are called soundlessly.
"Cheer for us now," someone behind us begs, "now is when
we need it."

My husband's face appears. He's crying. Caryl, why do you
suppose he's crying?

Caryl, give me your hand. We're almost there. See up
there at the top of the last hill.

"Drop your hands, ladies, drop your hands. You'll be
disqualified if you don't drop your hands. You're not
allowed to tie. Drop your hands, ladies."
We drop hands
and finish.
26 miles 385 yards 4 hours 17 minutes and 16 seconds.
It's over.

Epilogue

Three days later, sitting in an audience at Queens College,
having recrossed the 59th Street bridge
in a car to get there, I hear Tillie Olsen say, "And it
was the mothers who bound their feet, who had had theirs
bound before, and it was the mothers who sang songs to
them to soothe away the pain, to make up for woods not
walked in, streams not jumped over, and roads not
run down."
And then, only then, do I know my joy.

Back into This Body

Joyce Lombard

When I was a kid they called us tomboys
girls who braided their curls
got sweaty and dirty
climbed trees
lived in the branches beyond
the constructed structure daddy built.

Treading my way through years
of fancy dresses   marriages
pregnancies   school   nurturing others
I find my way back to the wild parts
of my woman's landscape
Discover hiking boots can stand
beside city pumps
Learn again to trust my body   walk into the fear
spend nights alone   with women   beside men
on forested lakes alive with sounds.

Trudging this narrow path
forty pounds of pack upon my back
Swimming close to the place where rooted trees
reach for clear lake water
I listen to the stillness
Catch my breath on the wings of a hawk

Find myself climbing the sky
toward home.

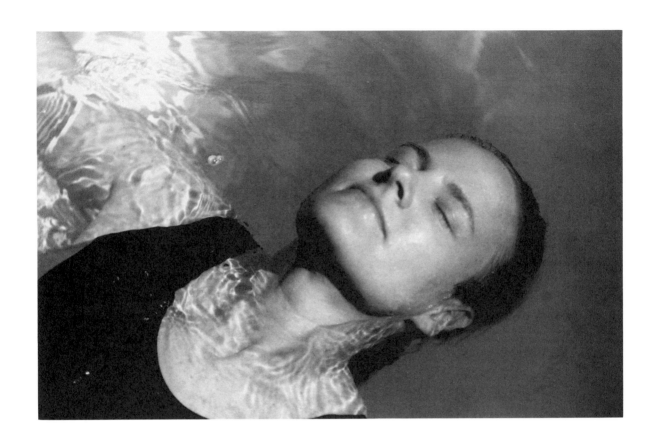

Return to Campus

Christine Swanberg

A passive student union.
A commune of heads glaze into the box.
Even during commercials, no one breaks
the electronic haze of soap operas.

Someone in a dorm insists on sharing music—
lyricless voices yelp and spit in goading offbeats.
The words sting like mosquitoes,
a surface itchy with short-lived poison,
scratched mindlessly with computer fingers.

Relics of past heroes hover—
insipid caricatures in posters.
Abbie Hoffman's wallet opens:
a fat, leathery slit.
A fake ID tucked in for validity,
polished with clean, crisp checks
of summer jobs and hardworking parents.

Timothy Leary smiles with perfect capped teeth,
and walks the aisles: a preppy saint
with a little gold chain on tanned neck.

They fill auditoriums to emptiness.
The curious sit in distant rows,
listen to paper words, unmoved—
satisfied with a little rush of the past.

Yet, campus women spring on thick, muscular legs.
Their calves become globes
in running shoes cushioned for giants.
Their nonchalant freedom wakens my slow steps.

Crossing the High Country

Amber Coverdale Sumrall

The narrow trail into Round Lake winds up and over a high mountain pass in a series of steep switchbacks. The morning air is cool and sharp; it stings when I inhale. This is my first backpacking trip since I lost my leg fourteen years ago in an auto accident. I climb slowly and methodically, not yet acclimated to the altitude. I wear a below-the-knee prosthesis on my right leg and a foot brace on my left. I am aware of every stone, every piece of wood on the path. One false step, one twist of my ankle or knee, and I would have to be carried out of the Sierra Nevadas. For leverage and balance, I use a gnarled branch of madrone as a walking stick.

I have been walking and practicing yoga for weeks in preparation for this. On my back is a day pack, stuffed with my sleeping bag and a dozen wool stump socks. A pair of field glasses for bird observing hang from my neck. My husband, John, carries forty pounds of gear on his back.

"You set the pace," he tells me, following several steps behind. "You'll get to flush the birds too." He has hoped ever since we met that I would someday be able to experience the high country and is prepared to do anything to make this possible. We will walk for five miles, then make camp.

I have known John over eight years. The fact that I am an amputee made not the slightest difference to him when we met. It does now though. When I limp around the house, steeped in self-pity and loathing my "condition" as he calls it, his patience wears thin. "Everything's conditional," he says, the way hippies used to say, "Everything's relative." John thinks I should have a hut to go to at these times, modeled on the menstrual huts of Native American women. A quiet, solitary place to reflect and heal. He refuses to indulge my self-destructive moods but will massage my foot, back, neck, legs, whenever I am in pain.

It is early morning in the Sierras, the sun has not yet crossed the snow-capped peaks. Robins and purple finches punctuate the silence with song. Across the valley, patches of snow are melting, becoming streams that feed Woods and Winnemucca Lakes.

Last week I had the screws tightened in my artificial foot and bought a new pair of hiking boots. At the last minute I decided in favor of my old, well broken-in work boots. As we climb up the mountain, my artificial foot begins to creak. So much for sneaking up on birds, I think, wondering if this leg is going the way of my last one.

Several years ago at an art exhibit, I found myself falling mysteriously in slow motion. I grabbed onto a table of leather-bound journals to stop my descent, but they tumbled down with me. I noticed that my foot was hanging by a thread from the rest of my prosthesis. It swung back and forth like a pendulum. A crowd formed in record time, unable to comprehend that this was not a flesh-and-blood foot. "Is she drunk?" someone asked, in response to my wild laughter at their horrified expressions. "Drunk or crazy," someone else replied, as I sat on the floor wondering how to escape the pandemonium. A fellow amputee, sensing what had occurred, pushed through the crowd and carried me to my car. It was worth the discomfort and embarrassment to see the shock register on all those faces as they stared at my rapidly swiveling foot. I felt as if this was my initiation into a secret, esoteric club. Able-bodied need not apply.

At the summit of Meese Pass we stop to rest. I gulp air greedily, attempting to make up for the reduced oxygen. The rising sun has illuminated the meadow below and for as far as I can see there are wild blue iris, bright yellow mules ears, and purple lupine. I remove my outer flannel shirt, change my stump sock which is wet and hot. I will have to change them every thirty minutes to prevent blisters and sores. They slip easily through the loop on my pack and will dry in the breeze while we walk.

Clark's nutcrackers dart from tree to tree, collecting pine nuts from Jeffrey pines as we enter a series of meadows threaded with tiny streams. I want to come back as a bird. To choose whether to walk or fly. It is no coincidence that my dreams of flying have increased lately; I have been so frustrated with the sheer effort of moving my body from place to place. It seems that as soon as my ankle recovers from tendinitis or my sciatica is in remission, my stump develops a painful pressure sore which necessitates hours of not wearing my prosthesis. Flying appears to be so effortless.

It is a rare occurrence when I'm not dealing with some imbalance in my body. Most of the time I am able to take it in stride and chalk up more writing time (sitting at my desk requires no great energy expenditure other than tremendous willpower). But on the bad days, I internalize anger and contempt for my body as if it were the enemy, plotting my demise.

When the simple act of walking down to my garden for tomatoes or squash irritates my ankle or stump or both, I become afraid and withdraw. The "how could anyone ever want to put up with me" mantra resonates through my head, and the familiar fear of dependency wells up to such an extent that I refuse to answer the phone or reach out to my friends. I clump around the house ranting and raving like a madwoman, and even my cats avoid me.

John and I stop at the headwaters of the Truckee River to wash our faces. Removing my prosthesis, I check for redness and bathe my leg. From this point it is all downhill to Round Lake, through subalpine meadows, then forests of red and white fir. Dozens of woodpeckers, warblers, lazuli buntings, and nuthatches flit overhead, and the rising warm fragrance of crunched pine needles beneath our feet permeates the air. Finally, we pass through a dense canopy of lodgepole pine to arrive in a beaver's marsh bordered by a quaking aspen grove.

"The lake's just beyond those trees," John says. "I'll scout the easiest way in. How are you doing?"

"I'm exhausted, ready to eat."

"Yeah, me too. It's the altitude."

He sheds his pack and disappears beyond the aspen grove. Unstrapping my prosthesis, I check for swelling or irritation. The air temperature is cool at this elevation, a critical factor. My stump is fine.

"There is no simple way down," John says on his return. "We have to make our own trail from this point. There are lots of rocks to climb over."

Slowly, we pick our way across the maze of granite boulders. This is extremely difficult for me, my artificial foot is not flexible, does not yield to the surface beneath it. It wedges in the small clefts between boulders. When we arrive, hand in hand, at our chosen campsite, there are no other people at the lake. We have the water, the birds, the fish, all the beauty of this place to ourselves. Above us are pinnacles of vertical rimrock, eroded into strange formations, lifting from the lake. A perfect nesting site for golden eagles and red-tailed hawks.

Two days ago, when John was working on our sauna, I told him I was ready to go to Round Lake, and he said he'd take time off. I first heard about this magical place from him; he'd been here long ago. My decision was not a conscious one. Rather, my body gave signals that it was capable, and I responded, trusting, as I have recently learned to do, in its innate wisdom.

Last spring when I was putting in my garden, I refused to stop digging when my stump began to hurt, needing to go beyond the pain, to "overcome" it. As a result, I was unable to wear my prosthesis for days afterward. Used crutches and a wheelchair.

After a short rest, during which several mountain chickadees and Steller's jays check us out, we pitch the tent and hang our food to keep it safe from bears and raccoons. Choosing the perfect rock overlooking the lake, we devour our lunch of hard-boiled eggs, trail mix, and bananas. It's true what John says, *anything* tastes gourmet after hours of hiking.

His sense of humor tends toward slapstick, but he has never hidden my leg as a practical joke even when he knows I am liable to ruin his morning on any given day by following him around the kitchen with a full list of grievances. When I kicked the basement door in, totally enraged after the third of three custom-made prostheses in one month didn't fit, he calmly stuffed the jagged hole with newspaper. Later, he transformed one of the prostheses into a planter, filled with forget-me-nots, for my birthday.

Tossing the last of the trail mix to the juncoes, we make our way down to a slab of smooth granite at the water's edge. John unpacks his fishing reel and baits a hook with silver lures to attract cutthroat trout. Shedding my clothes, I stretch out in the hot sun, close my eyes, and listen to the whir of the reel.

A week ago I was at Tassajara Hot Springs, east of Big Sur. Women of many ages and sizes lay naked together on the deck by the creek. I felt shy when I took off my clothes; even when I did not observe them looking, I felt their eyes on me, their unspoken questions. As I entered the steam bath with my friend Diana, who carried my prosthesis in and out (it's not waterproof) as I needed it, one of the women asked about my leg. When I told her about the accident, she took both my hands in hers, looked me in the eyes, and said, "Thank you for the courage and beauty you bring to this place."

I did not grow up loving my body. The messages I received, as an able-bodied Catholic girl in the fifties, were consistent in their negativity. My body was considered a temple of the Holy Ghost, on loan from God, to be held in trust like a gold certificate until I died. A woman was classified as virgin, whore, or mother. How to get from virgin to mother and still have a good time was a dilemma for many of us. I opted for becoming a tomboy.

Actually, it is a relief to be the square peg in a round hole. To defy the labels and stereotypes. To be the tomboy again. So that at Tassajara, when I sit among women, naked and vulnerable, it frees me to accept my body a little more.

Sliding off the rock into the icy water, I swim over to the beaver dam that we walked across a few hours ago, a bridge of aspen limbs, mud, and dried grasses. It appeared so fragile I couldn't believe it would support us. Water hyacinth pads float across the lake; lazily I glide among them as John lifts fish from the water. As the afternoon shifts to evening, we return to our clothes and gather wood for the campfire. John prepares dinner: panfried trout, rice, and cheddar-cauliflower soup. The stars appear, one by one, the Big Dipper directly overhead. We drink hot chocolate as the flames die down, relaxing into the serenity of this place. My entire body aches, but it is a good ache, muscles exerted to their capacity. As the moon rises, we bed down in the tent, sleeping bags zipped together, our bodies twined around one another.

The loss of my limb did not affect my sexuality. I decided after the accident, at age twenty-eight, that anyone who would reject me on purely physical grounds was not someone I'd care to be lovers with. Because I could "pass" as an able-bodied woman most of the time, it was often quite a shock for a potential lover to learn of my disability. I confess to a perverse delight in witnessing people's reactions over the years. John is fond of saying, "It's not how you're built, it's how you're wired."

Something wakens me in the night, a receding sound close to the tent like a large animal scuttling away through the woods. I imagine it is a bear, can't get back to sleep. There is always some fear to deal with, tangible or intangible. Ultimately, it is the fear of dying that permeates all the others. I believe that those who are most threatened by the disabled are those who do not acknowledge their own mortality. Those of us who are disabled are continual reminders of nature's random workings. I prefer to think of those who are not disabled as *temporarily* able-bodied. Sooner or later most of us will experience a major disability. Not many of us die in our sleep these days.

At first light I awaken again to the raucous sounds of a Clark's nutcracker picking through the ashes of last night's fire. It flies off with a small clump of rice. There are days when I feel like such a scavenger. Days when my stump retains water before my period, and my prosthesis will not fit properly. Days when my ankle will not support me. I am like the bird, searching for sustenance among the ashes. Sometimes I manage to pull something out: a book, a remembered chunk of advice, a phone call to a friend, the appearance of a special bird at my feeder, a poem that surfaces, or the stunning beauty of the day itself.

After breakfast of trout and eggs, and one last swim, we prepare for the long hike out. It is noon, very warm, and an uphill climb most of the way. I need to stop frequently to rest, drink from the canteen, change socks. It takes over four hours to reach our car at the trailhead. I allow my body to carry me slowly, to take the time it needs.

After the place where the mountain pass levels out and the switchbacks end, there is a wooden plank crossing a stream. Lush plants spring up on either side. The plants and herbs are unfamiliar but their fragrance is not: a blend of citrus, lavender, and sage. An image of my grandmother Nellie June's bedroom comes to mind. It is the way her room smelled when I visited. The mixture of sachet, dusting powder, and orange blossoms from her fruit trees outside. She has come from the spirit world to greet me here. Her words echo down the canyon, "Honey girl, if you listen to your own inner voice, you'll never go wrong." My grandma with her wisdom and Mohawk connections to the earth taught me to believe in myself. I silently give thanks for her blessing, for this crossing.

As John and I pull shoes, socks, dirty jeans off by the car, I am already contemplating my next adventure. I want to participate in the upcoming blockade at Concord Naval Weapons Station, a major distribution point for arms shipments to Central America. As a sanctuary activist, this is an issue close to my heart. Because I need my arms free, for equilibrium, I cannot allow myself to be handcuffed. A wheelchair is the only alternative. This means I will leave my prosthesis at home. I am afraid of being so vulnerable, so dependent on others. I am scared and uneasy, and I am going to do it anyway. For Nellie June, for all disabled women, for myself.

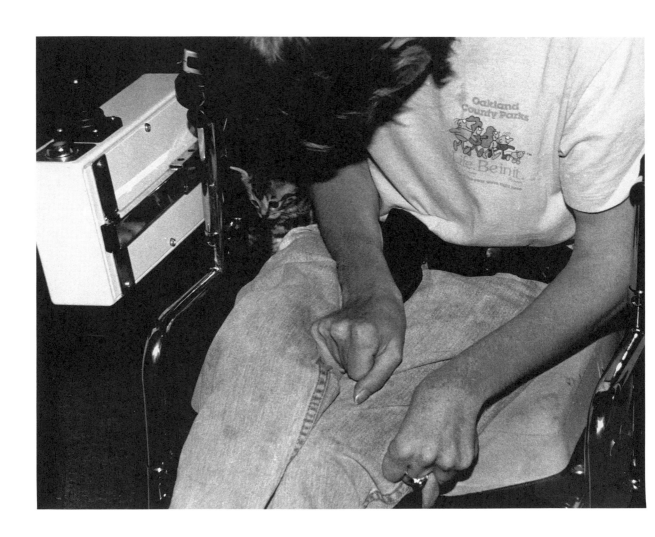

To My Body
Judy Clouston

I thought
you had deserted me
so I disowned you.

I hauled you
from place to place
endured
    your failures
administered
    your needs.

I could not
trust you.

Now I bless you for
adapting
    adjusting
        accepting

You move
in the water
as gracefully
as a mermaid.

Premenstrual Syndrome

Sharon H. Nelson

This is the time of the month when you find
your husband's a fool,
regret having children, wish
you had studied music, architecture, law, anything but how
to get the potatoes, green beans, roast, and rolls
all hot and on the table together.

This is the time of the month
when your patience has shrunk
to the size of a pea.

This is the time of the month you discover:
the house you live in is unsuitable;
you'd rather throw out the dishes than wash them;
you've always detested ironing.

This is the time of the month
when things you usually overlook
irritate you to screaming;
when things you don't usually notice
take on proportions that drive you to frenzy.

This is the time of the month
when you stomp
out of the house,
drive aimlessly round the city,
just to get away from the noise,
the electricity created by lives
rubbing up against each other,
and also,
to remember
the feel

of your own flesh
on your own bones.

This is the time of the month
when everyone's wary,
when they smile slyly and shake their heads,
as if only they knew the name
of the dis-ease that afflicts you.

This is the time of the month
when doctors are kind to you,
prescribe tablets and capsules and liquids and rest,
are in sympathy
with those who must
live with this anguish, this tension,
this unfortunate physiological response to a genetic program,
that seems to provoke
witchery, bitchery, shadow, and shades in
otherwise perfectly respectable folk.

What if
this is the time of the month
when your perceptions are sharpest?

What if
this is the time of the month when
the illusions you hug round you,
warm and comforting and thick as a rug,
flap in the chill wind of seeing
what actually is?

What if
this is the time of the month when
the normal, the usual, are revealed
as the lies you tell yourself
three hundred and thirty days of the year?

What if
this is the time of the month when
the tears you haven't time for well up, overflow,
and you know, as surely as you know
what time of the month it is,
that your husband's a fool,
you regret having children,
you wish to study music?

What if?

Spa

Anne Giles Rimbey

Women become all eyes
at spas.
They eye lines
and curves
against a golden mean
of blooming bust,
shallow abdomen,
and slender shank,
measure themselves
and then each other.

First person dominates
bold thongs,
pink spandex,
and Lycra bindings.
With eyes
painted wide
they stare with
Sumerian votive
concentration on
each other.

I wish they would just
get naked
in that lighted, mirrored
room in
endless reflections
of Rubens mounds
of breasts and arms and hips
and dance
as goddesses
with each other.

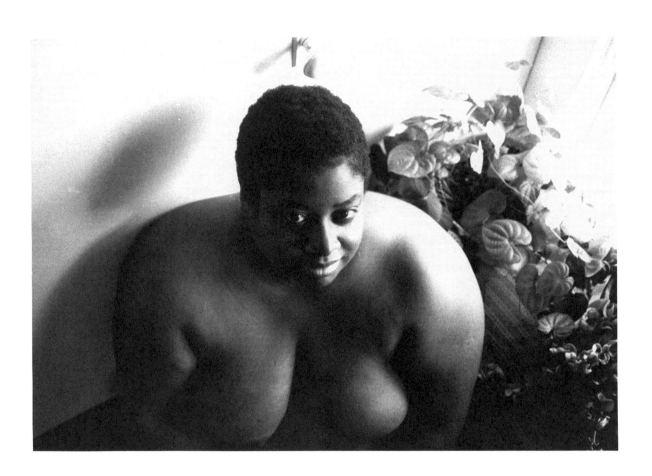

The Women's Side

Kim Ly Bui-Burton

The river comes here first.
It shapes a channel through rock
for itself, wide enough
to hold the rush of new water in spring.
This late in the summer,
what is wet barely covers
the spine of stones
in the middle, the curving ribbons
of weeds that wait hidden,
through autumn and ice,
until the touch of water
reveals them, again.

We bring only ourselves
down the narrow slope,
leaving layers of clothing
emptied inside,
on a row of polished wood pegs.
Do they remember
that once, they, too, were branching
green and connected, parts
of the whole?
My hand brushes the lowest twigs,
a tree across the creek
shivers. I smile.

Stepping slowly through heat-marbled
waters, I sink into the lap
of those velvet-skinned rocks
and long curls of grasses.
I had forgotten how to see myself
or another, without turning.

My body opens in warmth
and I can't look away, seized
by the beauty of bodies
around me: sloping breasts and rounded
carvings, the lower gardens
of moss and honeyed fruit.

O sunlight and sweat-shined skin:
I remember, I remember!

Figure Problems

Allison Joseph

Our eyes are trained to search
for flaws, to see our bodies
as problems that must be solved—

thighs too heavy, ankles too weak,
hips too wide to suit an ideal
we did not create—trained to see

each body part as fundamentally
troubled, astray. We learn to
conceal, not reveal, not to show

the weaknesses each magazine cover
prompts us to hide, shrouding
or starving ourselves submissive.

What if we were to disregard
the slogans that keep us indoors,
to shun the shame that marks us

imperfect, using our bodies
as we please, pleasure more
important now, more necessary

than perfection, our senses
stirred as we walk outside,
moving thighs and hips however

we want, moving forward in
steady rhythmic motion,
feeling power deep in

calves, knees, arms,
pushing as if against
current, yet still mobile,

aware of the air we breathe,
the persistent throb of our
heart, pulse. What if our bodies

were ours to master,
not the province of pills
or diet shakes, our own machines

to use however we wanted,
with variations here and there,
room for the slim and the curved

the angular and the heavy,
each one of us pushing the other
on, not holding anyone back.

Belly

Katharyn Howd Machan

This is the dance I dance for you:
red silk, gold coins, brass bells
making music through electric air
as you watch each step, each turn
of hand, ripple of hip and chest.

Though my dark-rimmed eyes never
look to yours, I move for you
as oud invites and drumbeat calls,
take your gaze deep into my blood
and find a wilder rhythm there
than any summoned alone. You say

let me be your skin and so I give
curve of all my nights, hot stars,
dawn silvering a thousand lakes:
I dance this dance of body's pledge
stronger than any spoken word.

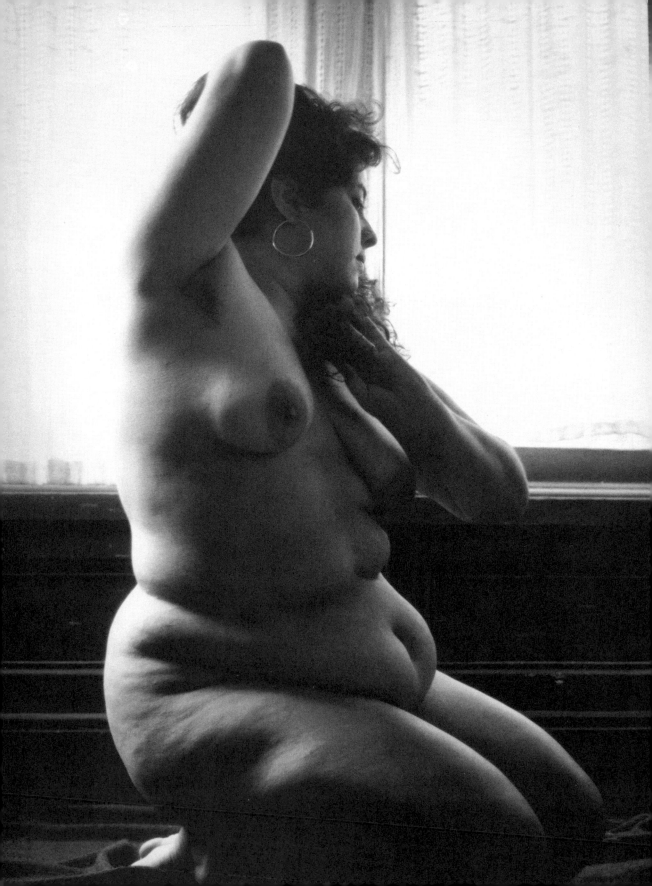

Contemplating a Breast Enhancement Operation

Rosaly DeMaios Roffman

My friend is taking a chance,
she sits like an apology in a chair.
I want to go to her and rock her
out of her decision, her dream of a pretty life.
Instead I boil up a cup of green tea
and talk not her, but me out of it.
We both sit drinking, eyes sending messages
into the hot of the cup. It is the puritan
voice of the Jew inside of me that says:
"God made you this way—be whole and grateful."

Stretch Marks

Laura Apol Obbink

You wear their names on your very body—
across breasts, curve of hips, once-smooth
span of belly, thighs,

your children's names imprinted on your skin.
Some women (whose selves live contentedly
in the bodies of others) call this

a badge of motherhood, a source of pride
which makes you, female, at last complete,
a hero of sorts. You see it

as the aching story engraved in flesh
of how you've changed, a sign to be read
like tree rings or strata of rocks,

line after widening line.

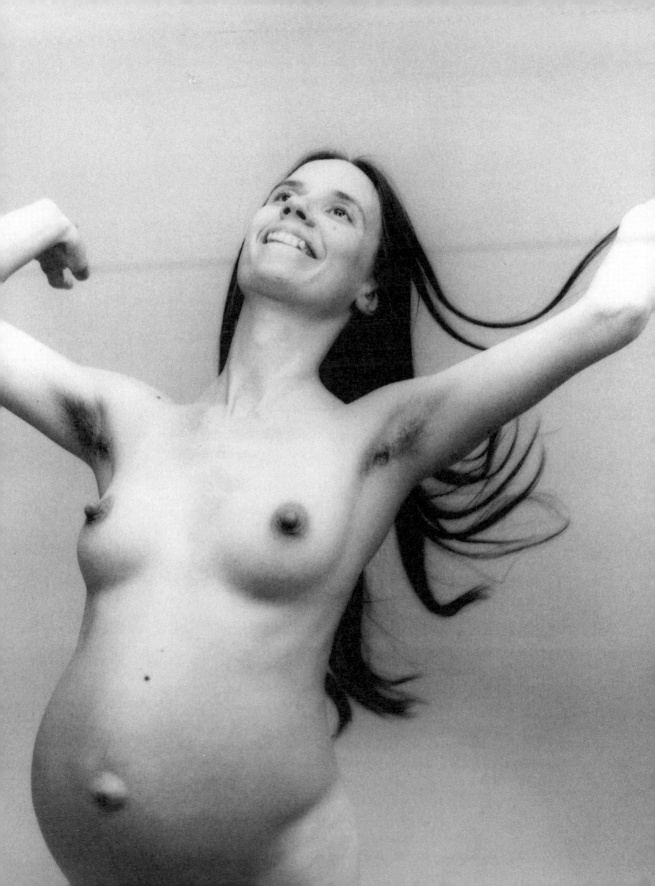

Seeing the Earth from the Moon

Maureen O'Brien

the contractions are gaining on me   catching me   I can't get up
the IV   I'm hooked to   the heart monitor   the fetal monitor
is wrapped around me   how can Tim stick with me
what if he leaves me   what if after this   he can't desire me
I look in his eyes   how can   he love me   who could
I have to pee   the nurse gives me a bedpan   I've never used one
Tim slides it under me   the contraction trembles   through me
"Should I turn around and not look?" he asks   I laugh "no" on
the bedpan as he jokes   "It's a new phase in our relationship"

the pain rises higher   I'm going to capsize   I am going under
and no one can swim   I am searching for air
where is my midwife? where   is Jill?   the pain   shovels me up
into the sky   sends me under   the tidal wave crest
Tim follows the contraction monitor   "OK,
you've reached the peak of it"   I slide down the wave
I look up in his eyes   I will drown if I look away   without his eyes
there is only the wave to grip

the contractions curl as regular as a whip   Tim instructs, "Slow your
breathing down! You're going too fast!"   who the fuck is he
he's a man   how the hell does he know how to swim this
he's never done it   I won't   surrender
how can I slow down when   this   slippery slamming

he breathes with me   gives me the pattern   I follow him   he is
right   I must slow down   cling to his rhythm
we breathe together   the pain   gathers me up   rolls over me
and the clock   how long has it been   six   hours already
the second hand goes around but the minute hand is   blocked
the clock   is a man

a wet washcloth   Tim leans over   cleans my face
how can he find me   how can   he see me   I am so far
down inside here   but they must see   he and Jill
call out my name   as if I am here   but how can I be
when the waves keep climbing   I'm going under

you   are not dilating   do you need the needle   should we get
the needle   we suggest the needle   here   he comes
you must drag your missing legs   over the edge   you must curl up
stay   very still   or else   a crowd gathers
who could love me   who   Jill sees me   down inside here
she searches for my hands   I hold a woman's hand
why haven't I   dangled all along   from a woman's hands
I don't care   who rides this needle into me
some man whistles "She's a real trooper"   I ride the waves now
I steer over them   on top

get cozy under the falling quilt   cry because you have no mama
let the pain   release you from its fury   shiver as you float over ice
see how those curtains just hang

Jill feels me with her fingers   "You're fully dilated!" she crows
this   baby is stuck   it's   too   big   I   have   to
get   it   out   can I push   have   to   push   so
push   lavender and yellow   explosions   have   to
push   I am nothing but a push   I am a woman
I am nothing but a woman bearing down

there is nothing else but bearing down
there is nowhere to go unless you   bear down   my husband
far away at my side   the nurses   far away at my feet
behind my eyes   red lasers explode

the baby has to move!   I am just a woman!   who am I now
who was I ever   a woman   can't keep a baby in like this!
I have to   get rid of this   baby   there is shouting
there is tension   the baby's heartbeat   too low!
call the doctor!   the baby must be turned   I see silver tongs
there   isn't enough room inside me   the pain grows larger
rounder   I am a push   I

look in the mirror   the baby's head is crowning   "That's your
baby's head! Your baby has hair!" the nurse sings   I don't give a shit
this fucking thing has to come out
I watch the baby disappear back inside   me   I knew it
it's never coming   I look down at the shouting
between my legs a doctor with a crooked ponytail   tongs steer into me
the roundness of a head   it's happening
a slice down the bottom of my   skin
I grip the roundness with a push   I push the roundness   it gets
bigger   rounder   fuller   people are running alongside me
stretching   the baby   so wide now   so wide open   the head
is sliding through me   the chorus swells
all the people dance between me   I am giving birth   we are being
born now   her head is out   I push   upon her body

all the people cheer   her body slides out   we are   all born

the baby rises in Jill's arms   I can hear again   rustlings above
the underwater sounds   I wait for words
"It's a girl!" Jill announces   a woman shouts "8:53 P.M.!"
my daughter   in flight   cries

"Is she all right?" I panic   the chorus sings   "She's great, she's
perfect!"   I fall off my elbows onto my back   I hear
someone else   crying   far away weeping   where is it   who
I realize   somewhere inside me   someone is weeping
but I can't feel tears   all I sense is lanterns   shining

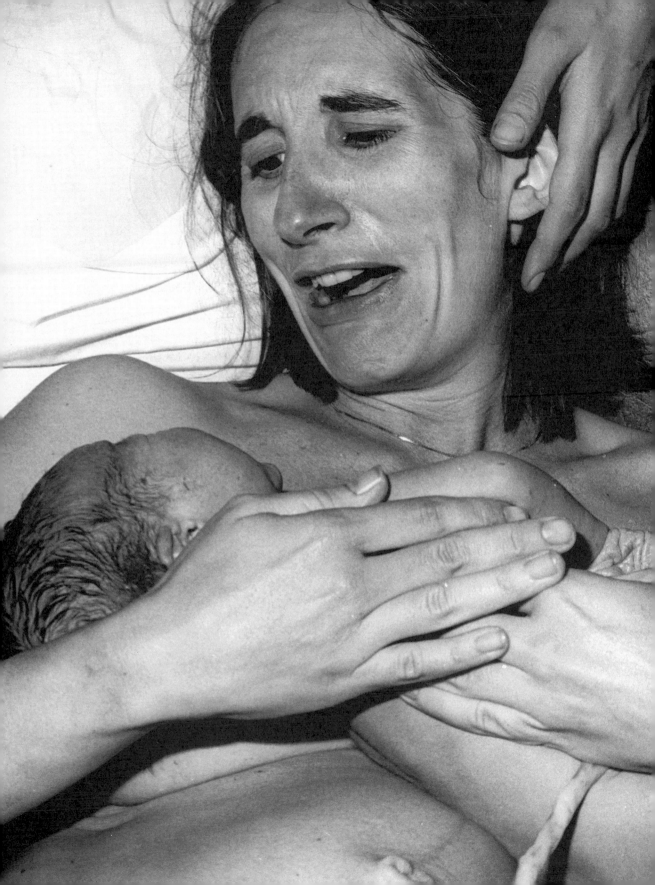

Tim keeps repeating   "She's beautiful, she's beautiful"
flashbulbs   pop   Tim asks, "Do you want to hold her?"
I hear her bare cries   high above me in the heat
I am suddenly nervous   I hear her circling   I open my arms
she is filling them   I am trembling   suddenly I hold her
she is crying and I have always loved her
she is my daughter and I am forever

her skin   I breathe it in   can you smell that   smells so sweet
don't you think   did you count her fingers   her toes
I'm counting   her hands rest   so beautiful   long tapered
fingernails   like a woman's hands   seeing her hands
I remember an astronaut quote:

he walked on the moon   he turned back to the Earth   (he said)
seeing the Earth from the moon   made him know there is God
made her know there is God

Breastfeeding at Night

Susan Eisenberg

I wouldn't mind so much
being your all-night café, if
after lingering over your drink
you went politely off to bed.

It's those nights when you
nurse one drink, then order another
    looking so *offended*
    your lips in tragic pout
when I suggest you've had enough

that make me consider
shutting the bar down altogether.

Forever

lu carter

I've said forever
I don't want kids
At least since I was twenty-two
And first aware that molding clay
Left unmolded gets dry and useless.

I load the noisy restless children
Of friends and family
Into my compact car
And drive to Peony Park,
Watch them run and scream
And ride their first roller coasters,
Win stuffed toys playing arcade games
I told them were a waste of money.
God, I sound just like my father.
My redheaded freckle-faced niece
Tells her parents she'd like ME
Named her guardian
Should anything happen to them.
I buy her soda pop
Give her my old Barbie doll clothes
Take her shopping and to the park.
She thinks I am wonderful.
I am
But not all of the time
Or even half of the time
It takes to raise a child.

The doctors tell me
Because I am still single and childless
I must live with pain for a few more years.
It is not ethical, they say,
To sterilize me—too young to know FOR SURE
I'll never want a child.
Are you 100 percent certain, he asks placing
The nonball end of his ballpoint pen on his lip,
That you won't marry and want a baby
Five years from now or even ten?
I see girl toddlers in the Dairy Queen dripping
Ketchup from their curly fries onto pink lace,
Subdue an urge to lick my napkin
And wipe their tomato-stained faces.
I stand in front of mirrors naked wondering
What I'd look like pregnant,
What a child pushed from me might look like.
I don't pretend to dislike children—
Only to decline the responsibilities of raising them.
I know my limits, I tell the doctor.

Handing me a year's supply of Ovral-28
And a prescription for Darvocet, he says
I just can't do it with a clear conscience.
Take more time to think about it.
After all
You'll have to live with your decision
Forever.

Tapping a Stone

Jane Schapiro

A coin, a shard, a pot, a lamp.
An archeologist explains how our world's
best secrets are the hardest to find.
Like him we believed in buried treasures,
thought we could, under the smooth terrain
of my naked body, find that one dark cave
where our waters run.
After all, we had the map, knew the rules,
charted the peaks and valleys,
and every evening
we'd find one more clue to convince us.
But somehow we were wrong,
the parched earth didn't yield,
the small brown smudge of the pregnancy test
signaled only a river gone dry.

Inside every stone a story,
the archeologist lectures on,
his fingers coiled around an ancient vase.
I watch him closely, as if he is a remnant,
a bit of unearthed truth
sifted out from a handful of dirt.
How I'd like to hold him up,
long legs, thick neck,
and say, "Here,
this is it, our proof."
Inside bones and brittle rocks
is the dust, the ground,
the breath of life.

Before Stillbirth

Barbara Bolz

The clouds, bloated and soon to labor,
    mock your death
    and me your tomb!
A bread crumb swells
in the sidewalk's moisture;
my stomach, too, expands and grows still,
quiet. More quiet
than even these windless trees
full and overburdened.

I imagine you've left my womb
to rock yourself in the crèche of this tree,
in the cradle of this uncommon fall.
You shake the trees with your cries
and others think it is the sound of rainfall
the wind mimics
in an ordinary autumn.

Stay in that tree
and in winter I'll watch you among
unfallen leaves, as you
rise higher and higher.
It will be a film I'll replay
of your naked body
rising over trees and beyond
this tree's children; you a weightless
stone that I love.

After Hysterectomy

Barbara J. Mayer

I travel the corridors
shuffling in fuzzy slippers
down barren stretches of slick tile,
hugging the walls for comfort,
a skater on wobbly blades.

A nurse meets my eye, looks away,
afraid I will lose my balance,
collapse in a heap.
I am a shipwreck listing dangerously,
a sailor washed up on an empty shore.

I hear a baby crying.
The sound grows fainter and fainter
until a door shuts with a whoosh
as if someone had whispered,
"Don't wake the children."

The Woman Whose Body Is Not Her Own

Anita Skeen

She is not herself anymore,
hasn't been since she stood before the mirror
in her own bathroom, holding
her own toothbrush, an ordinary
gesture, two days
later. She was lucky
to be alive, they all said, lucky
to lose something she didn't need,
not an essential foot
or a necessary hand.
They told her to rest.
They took her to dinner and talked
of the new kittens, the new boss
pestering like a small boy,
the small woman blessing them
from the corner booth.
The women across the table
were intact, might have lost a job
or a tennis match, maybe even
had lost touch with a son
or a good friend.
When she touched what was lost,
splayed her fingers across her chest
like a child cheating a peek
in a nightmare flick,
she heard the word *best*.
This is best, they said.
This is my breast, she tells the woman
in the glass, her hands cupped
like small graves

over the pale landscape, the shadow
of full moons. She feels the lips
of her first baby sucking
at air, sees him nested now in the crook
of his mother's life,
of this other woman's arm.

Gathering Morning Fire

Kaye Bache-Snyder

Thinking this may be the last time
sets my mind drumming
on what I had always meant to do.

So humor me and go in darkness
to the Colorado prairie
to watch this April day unfold.

We'll sit cross-legged on the sand hills,
lean back against the rolling wind,
and fill our lungs with aromatic sage.

We'll watch dawn's wildfire spread on the horizon,
the silhouettes of pronghorn flowing down the ridge,
and hear from bowls of darkness the dance of grouse begin.

I'll cradle the memory on another morning,
when a nurse comes to shave my thighs and stomach,
then rolls me pinioned on a cart toward the knife.

So go with me to gather fire from this dawning,
as it ignites the eastern sky, and pray
that as surely as the sun rises, so again may I.

Her Hair

Maggi Ann Grace

I was standing at the bathroom sink combing a new conditioner through my hair when my sister's face appeared in the mirror.

"Kara! For God's sake, can't you make some noise when you walk?"

She said nothing. We both stared straight ahead into the mirror, my arms still raised, the comb midstroke. I took a long look at our faces overlapping. While Kara's held a pale pewter cast, mine was tan, stretched tight.

"This light brings out the worst in you," I said, lowering my arms.

I waited for Kara to say something tart, or to pinch her cheeks to prove me wrong. She didn't move. I turned to face her.

"When you're done can we talk?" She was gone, as quickly as her face had appeared in the mirror.

I felt the teeth of my comb digging into my fingers, and I tossed the comb into the sink. Damn. It could only be one thing. Kara had been in remission for almost a year, after two gruesome rounds of chemo. She had announced back then, when she was released from the hospital the last time, that she would refuse further treatment "when the time came."

"Not *if* the time comes," she had said. Her doctor explained straight out that the odds against her multiplied with each relapse.

"I will not offer this, my body, as a battleground for chemicals and white cells ever, ever again." She'd waved her arms like a preacher and swung her legs over the side of her hospital bed.

Since her last "battle," Kara had gotten stronger, quit her job, and lived as she always had, every day a celebration. The rest of us seemed to forget the doctor's prognosis, that permanent remission was unlikely.

I fingered my wet, tightly wound curls to distribute them across my head. The conditioner hadn't relaxed them at all, but after watching Kara go bald it was a comfort to know that my hair was at least attached. Picking up the towel to dry my hands, I was grateful I no longer had to pick out the clumps of hair that stuck to the towels, the back of any chair Kara sat in, the shower wall. Bald was better.

I pictured Kara waiting to talk, probably sitting cross-legged on the living room rug in her moccasins. But I pictured her with a faint coral tint to her cheeks and those fistfuls of long dark hair down her back—hair she could french braid with pastel scarves woven in to match her outfits, hair she used to beg me to brush over the top of her head, upside down, while she stretched across the end of her bed.

"Come on." She would fold her arm up over her shoulder and pretend to stretch to the hem of her hair. "My arm isn't long enough to reach. And besides, I'm younger." But I suspected she enjoyed my envy—me, three years older and the shape of a telephone pole, with short, naturally frizzy hair the color of Dad's fruit trees in January. We were so opposite Mom used to call us her "salt and pepper girls." Dad called us Mutt and Jeff, whoever they were. When Kara and I argued about anything—clothes disappearing from my closet or one of us using up all the hot water—Kara would always manage to get in a dig about my hair. "There goes your head again, Julia, foaming at the mouth!" Right after Dad died, when we were all particularly irritable, she and I would get into it, and she'd say my hair was the color of death.

Kara would beg me to brush her hair, then bribe me with something I couldn't resist: like promising to cover for me when I stayed out late. So I brushed. And I watched the strands turn to silk, soaking up colors I never associated with hair. I secretly became addicted to performing this magic for her—and jealous, knowing those genes could have just as easily been mine instead; it was all in the way things got divvied up.

Kara was sitting in a wicker chair when I walked into the living room, not on the floor as I had expected. Her two best friends, Beck and Lyn, were perched at opposite ends of the sofa like two parrots in a cage. The three of them had been inseparable since Kara was first diagnosed.

"Hey, Julia," Lyn said.

Beck smiled a stiff little smile and nodded.

"Hi." I felt as relaxed as I did waiting for my calculus professor to pass out our final exam. I sat down on the rug and looked at Kara. She still had that dull metallic look about her, and I could no longer blame it on a fluorescent light in the bathroom.

"My liver's been complaining," Kara said, the way she might have said, "Let's grab a burger" or "I gotta pee."

I looked at Beck and Lyn to gauge their reactions. Nothing. Kara rarely mentioned her aches and pains, if she ever had any. I waited for the punch line to this liver joke. Nothing.

"Have you told Dr. Carrington?" I asked.

Kara nodded. "This morning my white count was at forty, platelets were only eighteen thousand."

I folded my hands and pressed, forcing my knuckles white. The last time Kara was admitted, her white count had been even lower than that. I tried to follow the bold zigzag pattern that sliced across the rug.

"So when are you going in?" I said.

Kara pulled on the spikes of new hair she'd grown. "I'm not."

"What? What the hell, Kara?"

Beck and Lyn scooted up to the edges of their cushions, as if I'd given a cue.

"Kara told us she wouldn't be readmitted, remember?" Beck said.

"So? When I fell off my bike and scraped my knee, I said I'd never ride a bike again too!"

"It's not the same." Lyn was up.

"Whose side are you two on?" I said. I looked at Beck, then back to Lyn. They looked steady, strong.

"Mine," said Kara.

I swallowed hard.

"Julia, I want you to understand," Kara said.

"I do! You're sick. When you feel bad, you've got to go get zapped again until next time. We all know that."

"I'll never be well, Julia," Kara said.

"You don't know that." I rose up onto my knees. "What about that guy who read his poems in the cancer ward last time? He'd been in remission for years!" I turned to Beck. She had been with Kara that day when the poet came.

"Different disease," Beck said. "His has a high cure rate."

I stood, thinking fast through a graph of percentages, white counts. "Those are numbers, Beck, just numbers! We can beat numbers!"

"I'm not competing," Kara said. "I quit."

"You can't."

"Julia, you don't have any idea how chemo makes me feel." Kara finally raised her voice to match mine. "It's worse than death."

"You can't know that either!"

"I'm positive." She sat back in her chair. "And each round postpones my dying."

I shook my head as if I could shake the thought away. Kara never stumbled over the words *death* or *dying;* other people did, but never Kara. "It's the only chance we've got, Kara—you have to try!"

"No, I don't."

"So die!" The fire rose in my face and lodged right behind my eyes. "How can I help?" I rocked back onto my heels. "You're young, you can't give up."

"I'm not. I'm making a choice," she said.

A choice. I thought about what few choices Kara'd had in the hospital. Tests, treatments, and when she looked like she was hanging on by a flimsy thread, more treatments. "Great guns," Dr. Carrington had called it. "We're going to hit 'em from all sides." Of course he meant the cancer cells, but Kara looked as if she'd been caught in a bloody battle which no one won.

"We're going to have a sweat before I die," Kara said, "and I'd like you there." She motioned to Beck and Lyn. "With us." Every eye was on me.

I looked at Kara. "What's a sweat?" I pictured Mom demonstrating my first spray can of Secret deodorant. Kara was seven and had been listening outside the bathroom door. When we opened it, Kara sang, "Julia's sweat is stinky. Julia's sweat is stinky." Mom went into this explanation of how horses sweat, but young ladies perspired. Kara and I never again said the word *sweat* without a laugh. And here she was wanting, of all things, a sweat.

"It's a purification ceremony where we recenter our spirits," Kara said. "A chance to unite ourselves before I go."

"Go? How can you can talk like that?" I said. "Kara, give it one more shot. Please."

Kara let the quiet in the room serve as her answer. I hated her—hated her for giving up. I recognized the black hollow feeling, that terrible feeling of not being able to hold on tight enough and losing what I wanted to keep. After Dad died, I convinced Kara that he'd be back, even after Mom told us he wouldn't. We hung onto that until we grew into the notion that he really was gone and we had to let go—the way we let go of the last kite we ever flew together at Winton Woods. Just the three of us. On purpose. Dad stood between us as we watched it become a real diamond in the sky.

"You want to do what to our spirits?" I asked, almost in a whisper.

"We want to join spirits," Kara said.

"Any blood involved? Needles?" I looked up to see if I'd pissed her off yet.

"Julia!" Kara rolled her eyes. "It's an Indian ceremony. We've done it a couple times already."

"Great."

"We heard about it last summer in Sedona," Beck said.

"No blood. No needles," Kara said.

"It'll feel like a sauna to you," Lyn said.

A sauna was the last thing I'd want before I died, I thought, but then some convicts order burgers and fries for their last meal. Kara had always been a little more—what? Experimental? I knew no one could predict the exact time of their death. We had no warning at all when Dad died. One morning we had a father, and by suppertime we didn't. And other people lasted years after doctors said they had only hours left, like old Mrs. Randall on the corner. But Kara would know. Right.

"If you'll bring Kara, we can set it up in the afternoon," Beck said. They were all looking at me again.

"Bring her where?" I had pictured them huddled in someone's steamed-up bathroom, writing on the mirror.

"We've been using the old Cedar Fork campground along the river," Kara said. "No one ever goes up there since they built that new bridge."

If Kara was that close to dying, she wouldn't want to go anywhere, much less to some powwow. And besides, Mom would be here by then. I had promised to call her when Kara got worse. I was safe.

"Die any way you want."

That night I dreamed we were all sitting around a campfire in lawn chairs fanning ourselves. Mom, Dad, Grandma, and Pops, even Dr. Carrington. But I had Kara's hair. And it was so long that I spread it out over my legs and stretched it to everyone around the fire. They all took hold of an end, the strands ran right through the flames, but it never caught. It looked like a maypole and like the huge hashish pipe I saw in the middle of some guy's dorm room my first year at State, with a tube to reach to everyone perched around the room.

But Kara caught me off guard five days later when she announced that the sweat would be that night. She'd been lying down a lot, eating even less than she usually did, even refused beer and wine, but she looked about the same. Gun metal grey.

"This whole thing's a lousy idea," I said.

"I'll take a cab."

"You're weaker."

"Are you refusing?"

I thought about refusing. About seven o'clock Kara and I headed toward Cedar Fork in my VW bug.

"Remember cutting Sunday school to come skinny dipping up here?" Kara said.

"Yeah, my memory's still intact." I glanced over at Kara. She had slumped down to rest her bare head against the seat. Her eyes were closed. I realized I hadn't called Mom.

"You OK?" I said.

"Yeah."

The bobbing of her head against the seat seemed violent; the new sprouts of hair were hardly the padding of the head of hair she once had, actually not so long ago.

"I don't have a pillow," I said, taking a quick look in the backseat. I grabbed an old flannel shirt. "Here, bunch this up under your head."

Kara raised her head up and wadded the shirt into an odd shaped tuft.

"You don't look comfortable," I said. "I can take you back home."

"No."

We reached a clearing at the top of the hill in only a few minutes. The trip had been quick, and I was grateful for Kara's sake. There were a couple of cars parked along the road, so I stopped and backed up in front of the first one to shorten Kara's walk.

A log fire was blazing in the center of a campsite only fifty feet away. It gave off such a blinding circle of light that the encroaching trees and scrub oak seemed to be hiding in a backstage darkness. Off to the left stood a teepee-shaped structure made of drab blankets. One of Kara's friends was carrying a rock the size of a basketball toward the fire. Then I saw Beck emerge from the teepee carrying a shovel. She speared the ground with the shovel and walked toward my car.

"A purifying ceremony, isn't that what you called it?" I said to Kara, turning off the ignition. "Looks like some tribal scene in *National Geographic*."

"You're foaming at the mouth, Julia," Kara said. "I said no blood, didn't I?"

When I glanced over, Kara's eyes were still closed.

I got out to meet Beck on the other side of the car. The night was as dark as it ever gets with a full moon—a Halloween sky, light dancing between cloud strips and evergreen branches into shadows on the ground. Beck's body was streaked in light.

"Perfect timing," Beck said.

I pressed my body flat against the car door and whispered so Kara wouldn't hear. "Some sauna."

Beck touched my arm. "It's what Kara wants. Let's get her out of the car." I stepped aside, and Beck opened Kara's door.

"Think you could give me a hand?" Kara asked from inside the car.

I helped her out, and she looped one arm around my shoulders and one around Beck's. "Thanks," she said faintly. She was weaker, I could tell that, but hardly ready to die. She couldn't be. She had walked out to the car, we'd been talking, and she became strangely calm. Was anyone ever ready? What if Dad had had a chance to prepare a little?

My face felt seared by the heat as Beck steered us around the bonfire toward the teepee. We ducked under a blanket flap that had been pulled aside as an entrance. Lyn and another one of Kara's friends were digging out a deep hole in the center. Lyn stopped and came over to hug Kara. She motioned to a blanket and a tall pillow off to one side, and Beck and I helped Kara over to it. Inside, away from the fire, it was cooler, but the raw smell of fresh earth and perspiration was thick and sour like a locker room after one of my muddy softball games.

Lyn laid her shovel down. "I think that'll do it," she said.

Without any apparent signal, the women came in and stood around the hole.

"We need to get our clothes off," Kara said. Kara looked relaxed against the pillow. I started to sit down beside her.

Beck put her hand on my shoulder. "Julia, you'll probably want to slip yours off too. We'll go down to the water after this."

Everyone seemed to know the rules. This was what Kara thought was the end of her life, and her friends were parading around like it was a laboratory experiment, ordered by protocol.

Kara eased her sweatshirt off over her head. Beck helped.

"Julia, I'd like for you to be part of this," Kara said. "Won't you?"

It wasn't that I minded getting naked. I was used to team showers. How did Kara have the energy for all of this? She could stretch out on the sofa at home. She could be comfortable. Let Kara have her little ceremony, then I'd drive her home. I'd put on some Windham Hill tape. I'd drive around the ruts.

I slipped out of my jeans and T-shirt.

Two of the women brought in rocks on shovels from the fire outside and dropped them into the hole. The temperature rose almost instantly. The air became heavy, thick. The earth spit, and the sound of it made me jumpy. No one else seemed nervous or afraid, especially Kara. There was no wailing, none of those empty stares that seem to bore right through a person's face, like the faces I had to sit and look at the night Dad died, when all of the relatives were sitting around our living room.

Beck lit a couple of candles. Another woman pulled the flap down to seal the teepee. She sprinkled water from a small bucket onto the rocks, and patchy clouds of steam lifted above us like tufts of cotton stretched too thin.

I felt light-headed. "I should take you home," I whispered to Kara. "You're not strong enough for this heat."

Kara cocked her head to one side. The candlelight patterned her forehead and chin with tiny crescents of white light.

"If you get too hot, you can go out and cool off. I'm fine."

She was fine. She was dying, but she was fine. The way Mom said that Dad insisted he was fine when she found him, lying in the driveway beside the old Rambler holding his chest, repeating, "I'll be fine," over and over again while they waited for the ambulance. In the rain. Mom didn't dare move him. It rained hard all day that day. And by sixth period when Mom reached us at school, Dad was dead. Just like that. No good-bye, no nothing. We even ate sloppy joes and orange wedges in the cafeteria, just like normal. Never knew anything was different.

Sweat trickled down my cheeks, my neck. The hissing and sputtering of water on the rocks grew louder. My eyes and nose stung.

I turned to Beck, my heart wild. "This is suicide!"

"It's just like a sauna." Beck's voice was calm.

"Saunas are for healthy people, strong people."

"I won't ever be healthy." It was Kara's voice, delicate. "Julia, may I have it my way?" And then in the tiniest voice, "Please?"

I reached for my jeans.

"I need to do this," Kara said, "and it needs to be tonight." She closed her eyes. I knew she was hurting, though pain never showed in her face.

Never had. Not even when the chemo turned her inside out. When she was lying in that hospital bed, her skin more the color of cold ash than of anything alive, the only emotion I could read was humiliation. Never fear. Never pain. I stared into my sister's face, into the eyes of someone who wouldn't, who couldn't have it her way for long.

I inched myself over to let her lean against my arm. Her body was limp. Her hot face puddled against my bare skin. She was getting weaker by the minute. She smiled.

Beck slipped her hand into mine and a low, slow chanting spread around the circle of Kara's friends.

> We are the flow,
> we are the ebb.
> We are the weavers,
> we are the web.

A twig was stuck against my thigh. I looked up, and, between gusts of steam and smoke, I saw the moon perfectly framed by the hole in the teepee, so full it looked more like the sun. They repeated the words of the chant over and over until it became a simple rhythm.

A woman on the other side of the teepee spoke about her life before this one, of her mother who died giving birth to her—somewhere in a hot climate was all she knew. "I'm going to get to Alaska someday," she said, "or at least someplace cold."

Weird talk. I strained my eyes to see the uneven chain of arms as everyone joined hands. Nipples, like a dozen terrified eyes, slick shiny skin. Sweat sprinkled their faces like shattered diamonds in the mottled light, flickering candlelight, a column of light from the moon—it reminded me of Dad camping out with us in the backyard when we were little, telling ghost stories with a flashlight under his chin.

Beck started talking about Kara's spirit, of cleansing, joining—words I'd associated with the Jesus freaks on campus. More rocks were brought in from outside. Lyn placed some stems of dry weeds on top before sprinkling more water, and the steam rose in such a quick curtain that her breasts seemed to disappear, leaving her head afloat. The weeds were probably healing herbs—Kara had books in our kitchen about herbs and natural remedies—though no one had mentioned this sweat thing as an attempt to make Kara well. The smoke carried a pungent odor now, sharp in my nostrils.

I wanted to leave, to fill my lungs with a rush of the cool, easy air I knew was just outside. But I couldn't leave Kara, not like this. I put my arm around her shoulders, and her body relaxed completely against mine.

There was more talk around the circle of connecting to Kara's spirit, of harmony, of nature, of being together again in another life. I felt Kara's body slip against mine. She raised her head up higher onto my shoulder, then leaned it to the side again. "Thanks for being here with me," she said—exactly what she used to say when she let me crawl into bed with her after the funeral.

She'd wake up about the same time every night calling out in her sleep, "Don't close it yet. Don't close it!" Kara's nightmare was the same for months—of the funeral director closing Dad's casket before she got there to see him. Just the way it really happened, except I figured out that in her dream Mom never made them open the casket back up. I was the one who finally realized what was missing in her dream. So when I climbed into Kara's bed for the last time, and she finally closed her eyes, I painted the end for her.

"Here comes Mom," I whispered in her ear, stroking her hair back off her forehead. "See her go over to that tall, skinny man in the black suit, the one walking toward the door in the corner? She's telling him to open that casket back up. He's looking up with that sickening smile, where his lips tuck up over his gums. Remember his smile, Kara, and his shiny head? You said it looked like a wet beach ball."

"Yeah. But it wasn't that big, was it?" She had stopped sniffling by then. "Thanks for being here with me." But I didn't stop.

"Keep your eyes shut," I said when she tried to look at me. "So here you come running in from the side door with Grandma, and I pull one of those folding chairs up to the casket so you can see real good. The funeral home guy lifts the lid; you climb up and look in. You get to look as long as you want."

Now I looked at Kara sitting beside me and saw her in that casket, but with her eyes open. Something let loose inside me, like breaking through the cloud of a fever, and I knew how afraid I was of losing her. I watched Kara's eyes scan the circle of her friends. She paused at each face and seemed to reach with her eyes. She didn't exactly nod, but they connected, that was clear.

"Take me home?" she asked, when she had completed the circuit. Her breathing quickened to short catches of air. I looked around to see who was still talking, but the images I could make out were all the same, of slick bodies leaning into shadows, like a garden of broken iris on a hot night.

I grabbed Kara's clothes and my own, and put them in Kara's lap. Beck didn't try to stop me when I lifted Kara and stood to leave. "What about going to the water?" I asked Beck. "Does she need that?" Kara felt lighter than I had expected.

"Kara's done what she came to do. She wants to go home."

I headed toward the doorway, and the chant continued. *We are the flow, we are the ebb . . .*

The air outside felt like rubbing alcohol in my lungs—cool, almost painful. Beck and Lyn followed me to the car and helped get some of Kara's clothes back on over her damp skin. I shivered—my arms and legs were like dotted swiss—solid goose bumps. They positioned her in the car while I dressed quickly. Beck kept weaving her fingers among Kara's, back and forth, finger by finger, like a current.

"Don't they want to say good-bye?" I said, looking back at the teepee.

Beck looked up at me. "We did."

Kara did seem content, complete. This was for real. I had to concentrate on getting her back home. I didn't want to be out riding around when Kara took her last breath, "in this life," as she always added.

I remembered the time about a year after Dad died when my mother found a book of Kara's under the front seat of the car, a flaming pink cover, the title something like *Life After Life* or *Life Between Life*. She wagged the book in the air, then ran into the house. At the supper table that night, she had calmed down and announced that she was sure we knew that life was here and now. "No second chances in this game." Kara hadn't argued with her.

I put the same flannel shirt under Kara's head again and started the car. Her limp body curved into the seat. I doubted she could hold her head up if she had to. The sweat had made her worse. I wanted to get her home, into bed.

"You OK?" I asked as easily as I could, the car bouncing over the deep ruts in the road. When Kara didn't answer, I said nothing more on the road back to the apartment.

I pulled up and parked in front of a cluster of pine trees and found myself repeating the chant—*We are the flow, we are the ebb. We are the weavers, we are the web.* It was exactly how Kara behaved, as if she could weave her life, and now even her own death, into her own design.

I managed to get Kara out of the car and carried her into the house. I lay my sister on the sofa draped with Grandma's comforter and went into the bedroom to grab Kara's hairbrush, a new soft-bristled baby's brush with chimes hidden in the handle—my joke when her hair started to come back in. I knelt beside her and brushed her hair, wishing I could silence the tiny bells, then massaged her head with my hands. Her head felt small. Kara opened her eyes, groped for my hand, and smiled. I could see her right eye had filled with bloody streaks.

Her eyelids closed, and her lashes lay in tiny dark triangles. Her breathing was still quick, short gasps of air when her grip on my hand loosened. The first time she'd let go of anything in many months.

I called Mom and told her to hurry, that Kara had gotten much worse. I knew I would never tell why. She would never believe Kara had wanted it exactly that way. Kara's breathing slowed to almost nothing with miles between each breath.

I finally heard Mom's car pull up, and she rushed in the back door calling Kara's name. When she saw her on the sofa she ran to her and laid her head to Kara's chest.

I walked outside to sit under the huge pine tree with the wide opening in its skirt—just like the one Kara and I used to sit under all bundled up in matching snowsuits. We'd crouch down, holding onto each other so we wouldn't tip over, and watch the snow fall around us like a white beaded curtain just beyond the boughs. As I knelt down in the pine straw, the hairbrush jingled like tiny chimes far away. Kara and I always felt safe behind the loose weave of the branches while all along we were right smack in the center of the storm.

Joan Has Her Ears Pierced

Bernice Rendrick

Beauty bombards us from wherever it can
    —Hortense Calisher

My friend Joan comes
wearing a black tam, a silver
teardrop dangles from one lobe.
You know, she says, it's something
to look at besides this bald head.

We talk of the shape of skulls,
her own, bare, frightening, a closure
over the ticking brain. How can we
make art of hair that falls in clumps?
Her blond braid of the sixties gone,
gradually cut by demands to spare lines.
But distinctive. She'd trim her bangs
a bit crooked or clip in a new fillip.
Now this skull grows fuzz, rejects it
as chemo shaves the head again,
deepens the patina of pain.

But she has made art!
Somehow, sick or well, every day.
It's on her plate and she eats it.
From under her ear it signals.
In her journal. Watercolor veils
do filmy dances, oil paint slides
with assurance over the bleak canvas.

It's me who loses concentration
as Joan loses her hair. It's me
who is having trouble
making art of this.

Hearing

Jeanne Lohmann

The sounds are never clear. They dance
a still perfection out of reach, and all
the straining forward will not teach
the ear that hears approximate. Interpret
as we can, we make a leap of faith, disguise
the fear of ridicule, laugh at ourselves
and take the strange noise in,
creating language from mistake.

Else otherwise we break our hearts against
this garbled world, confused and isolate
shut out the little that remains,
communicate despair, give in to loss.
Translation saves us here, who find the word
holds true, a way would clarify life sounds
toward sense, and from distortion shape
the human music, make the meaning new.

To My Eyes

Mary McGinnis

I write to my eyes out in the high desert. I write to them when I'm half asleep, so that true dream images will slip off my fingers. What I tell them comes from the inland sea of tossing dry grasses and yucca stalks out in a field of dusty cholla and juniper bushes. Dreams and images don't lie. Images from the weeds and pack rat nests float up from inside me. They illuminate and warm me, the way the sun does, reflected off the glass in winter.

I used to think my eyes were the problem. Once a rehab counselor said that people might look at them and feel uncomfortable. Kids sometimes said they looked funny. They'd come up to me and ask me what *was* wrong with my eyes, and at one time I actually thought something was wrong with them. Lately, I've come to know that my eyes have done no harm. In the right setting, light glints off them, and they sparkle. Usually they're neutral as an arroyo. I've come to like their softness.

It's what I've told myself about my eyes that's been the problem. I've been on guard, planning my route through my life, preparing for every contingency so that having eyes that do not see wouldn't matter. I plan so I can feel grounded. In my waking life, I want to be perfect. I'm alert, I travel light, I make a mental circle around my possessions. I don't take more than I can carry on my back or in my arms. It's only in dreams that I don't pack everything I need, forget to bring the name and address of the hotel where I'll be staying, and wait for a drunken passenger to bring me my suitcase. It's only in my dreams that I'm in a bus station without a clue to where I'm going, a quarter for the pay phone, or my cane.

Once, distracted by poetry and daydreaming, I left my backpack containing my slate and stylus and scratch paper up at the snack bar at Bandelier National Monument. When I got home and realized what I had done, I was disgusted with myself. I thought about how my writing implements could be thrown in the trash by mistake forty miles from home. There must be something wrong with me to have forgotten them. But I had been betrayed by my mind. My eyes had nothing to do with it.

There have been times I have let myself go, gotten swirled around and transported by the liquids of myself: great sex, torrents of words, pinnacles of sound. Sometimes I can do it; I can step back from my mind, and the voices from the past talk on and on in my head without me. I'm there in the moment like a cholla, there being wherever I am, doing whatever I am doing. I'm like my eyes then. I'm full of emptiness and light, opening the wind of now. I am there; I am what I am.

Menopause Poem

Sue Doro

getting older
smiling through forty-seven years
I cook eggs for breakfast this morning
taking a necessary day off from the factory
I bite into my toast while thumbing through
Our Bodies Ourselves
chapter seventeen
"Menopause"
then I have to go the bathroom
and get my partial plate
that I left in its little blue plastic box
soaking overnight in baking soda
in the cabinet under the sink
because without all my teeth
the toast in my mouth
is too difficult to chew
and I laugh with myself
seeing myself holding a piece of bitten toast
reading about menopause
and hunting for false teeth
because what I'm looking for
in chapter seventeen
is how to best keep on making love
with a vagina that tends to dry a bit
and the good old *Our Bodies* book
answers with
saliva
KY jelly
and a loving partner
so as soon as I finish my eggs
I'm on the way to the drugstore
to get the one I don't have

This

Ann Menebroker

You get out of bed
solemnly naked
and lumber somewhere
out of sight.
The house
is a mystery
the way
it swallows
whoever leaves
warm sheets.
Lying here
in my old
bare skin
I think
how I love
the sight
of unclothed people
going about
the business
of love.
Everything else
is so ruined;
the room, the landscape
the world.
The way to stay
beautiful
is to avoid
mirrors
and look only
at those
who truly
love back.

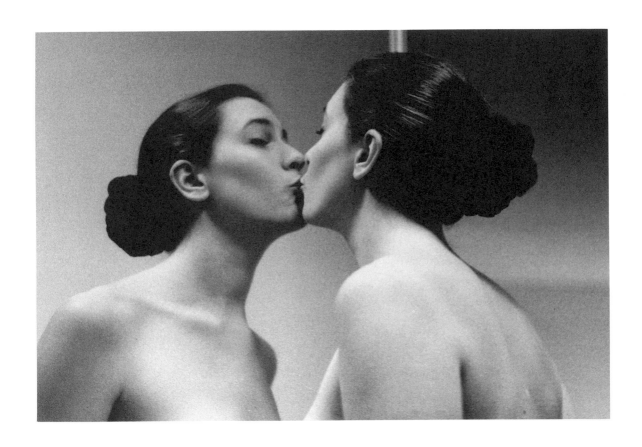

After Reading Mark Strand's "Courtship"

Beverly Voldseth

Today it takes the form of fever
and although I have said all day
and yesterday too
that I am getting Lizzie's cold
and although my nose runs
and my body has that crisper-than-tissue-paper
feel, at 3 P.M. I know it is simple lust.
I should have known when
I caught sight of my mirrored breasts in the morning dark
round and full and reaching
that desire was building in my veins.
And later innocently working through a stack of mail
every magazine fueled it
poems and stories kerosene on the blaze
sending my hand up under my sweater
my breasts under my hot palm
cool and firm needing a mouth.
But lust is never simple.
Oh, I know, simply, what I can do about it
alone in the house all day
no lover I can run to.
I know what I can do
and then it's done.
But it's not done.
The skin still burns for touch
ear wants teeth and tongue
nose wants odors of bodies mingled
and the brain still wants, wants, wants.

Better Than Sex

Keddy Ann Outlaw

The nurse-teacher-artist
drives home at noon.
She takes off
her stockings
and lies on the sofa
in a meditative nirvana
her mother called a nap.

If you asked her just then
she would tell you
such silence
is better
than sex.

Better than
the better-than-sex cake
someone always makes
for holiday parties,
the one with whipped cream,
pudding, cherries, sponge cake
and gooey chocolate.

Afterward, she
wonders—can anyone
identify the pillow crease
on her face, that scar
of a lunchtime assignation
with loose and lovely self.

To Women Who Sleep Alone

Amy Uyematsu

my mother doesn't understand a world with no man in it
tells me I waste too much time
forgets I used to spend hours playing by myself.

I don't tell her what sleeping alone is really like
the sweet oils no one but me can rub into my skin.
I look at my body again
no longer as pretty
all the young men I've sent away
will not be coming back.

lately my body's scent fills every room to smother me
I wonder if any man can still enjoy its taste
a darker odor.
every month my blood flows harder
an ache building within my thighs
a real part of me dying—
I want to let in the smell of trees and wind after it's rained.

there's a small grey bird outside my house
who keeps building
her nest with pine needles.
every evening the wind scatters her work
but she returns the next day with new twigs
determined to make a home here.

I'm not one of those women
who can make up their minds
just like that
to find a man again—
something my mother never taught me.

men have always come to me
asked me to dance
I'm not sure how to bring them back in.

sometimes I take a small branch of asparagus fern
twirl it around and around—
a light green fuzz powdering my arms.
then I curl my hands under my breasts
reassured by the softness of skin
remind myself this is enough for now—
my thin hand pausing on the shoji door
running my fingers along rice paper and wood—
a woman opening to the sound of rain.

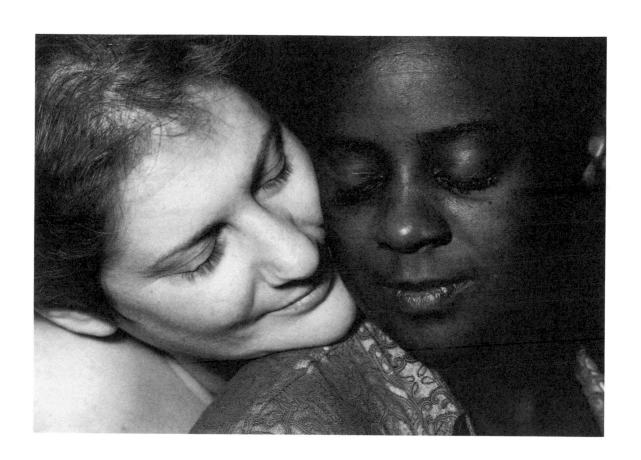

The Pier

Michele Moore

At 2 A.M. the front door opened, and Cecilia sang out in full voice, *"Piágni, Piágni!"* In the bedroom, Amanda lay on the floor trying to get a suitcase out from under their bed.

"Are you all right?" Cecilia rushed to Amanda. "There's blood on your shirt, did you fall or—"

"Blood? Where?" Amanda twisted around to look at a spot on her hip. "Hey, how about grabbing that brown suitcase for me?"

"In a minute. Roll over a little more."

Cecilia smelled of Eternity, her newest perfume. Amanda loved the fragrance on her and told her so as she rolled to her stomach.

Amanda could feel Cecilia's hands on her back, though not much below her hip bones. Amanda wasn't really numb below the waist, it was more like degrees of vagueness—knowing when she was being touched but not precisely where.

"You should have waited for me to help you pack."

Scratches didn't faze Amanda. It took a deep cut for her to feel pain in her legs.

When she was eight years old, Amanda fell through a rotten board on a fishing pier in Florida. The doctor had said she was lucky because the bones she broke in her spine were low enough that muscles in her arms, hands, and much of her back were normal. Now, at thirty-one, her arms and upper back were quite muscular. Her body frequently evoked the response, "You seem quite athletic," from people who might have only seen her reading a book or eating in a restaurant.

"Just a scrape. Here. Can you see?" Cecilia handed Amanda the mirror, then, as if overcome by exhaustion, closed her eyes, slumping back against the bed and into her wild sea of electric-red hair.

"Great finale tonight. Next season you'll get a solo part. I can feel it."

"You always say that. Anyway, I'm taking an audition in Seattle in August."

"Seattle! With all the rain?" Amanda pushed herself up onto her elbows.

"And steep hills, too. Don't forget any of the standard objections."

Amanda pulled her oversized pajama shirt down before lifting herself back up into the wheelchair. "I love opera. Its women are sacrificed so beautifully that we forget our standard objections."

"Oh, *please!*" Cecilia rose to her feet and, with a haste that screamed anger, began to help Amanda pack.

"Take Desdemona. Not only is her spouse murdering her, but she has to sing that final aria with her head hanging over the edge of the bed." Amanda shoved a hardback book into a plastic bag, glancing to see if Cecilia had smiled or snickered or done any other gesture to ease the pain of their conversation.

Cecilia dropped a stack of Amanda's T-shirts into the suitcase with dramatic emphasis. "I don't know why I'm helping you pack this thing. You won't be able to manage it alone."

"The suitcase?" Amanda smiled, then tossed a bathing suit at Cecilia.

Cecilia sat down, becoming eye level with Amanda. "How wide is the bathroom door in your hotel room?"

"I've stayed there before!"

"You were eight years old! Stop being foolish."

Amanda closed the suitcase and wrestled it down to the floor. "You want to be my guardian angel?"

"I don't want you to go by yourself."

Amanda wheeled close to the bed, giving in to a spark of hope. "Then you're coming?"

"You know I can't miss the Santa Fe festival. What about your parents? They live on the water. Or wait for me, and we'll go next year."

"Forget it. I've been waiting for you. And listen, I stay alone here plenty. I manage all right. Good thing, too, considering how much you've been around lately."

"We were talking about you and this insane trip. But if you want to change the subject—"

"I'm going to Florida by myself, and that's that." Amanda flung her hips onto the bed from her chair. Cecilia grabbed her robe from behind the door and left the room.

From the kitchen came the sound of eggs frying, and now and then, her sweet voice singing out, *"Piágni, o misera, piágni!"*

Predawn flights had the advantage of not being crowded. Even with

Cecilia, traveling was tedious; without her, Amanda lacked the emotional insulation from flight attendants as they transformed her into a sack of potatoes, lifted her onto a dolly-type thing, pulled her down the plane's narrow aisle, then, barely smiling, heaved her up and into her seat. There, without choice, Amanda stayed, trying not to dwell on this particular confinement until the plane landed.

Exhausted by the combination of fear and no sleep the night before, Amanda waited outside the baggage claim area for a cab driver willing to take someone in a chair.

Being the oldest city in America, St. Augustine was home to "The Oldest" of many things. Ponce de León's Taxi, The Oldest Taxi in America pulled up to the curb. The portly driver, dressed in full Castilian finery walked briskly toward Amanda. His dark, precision-trimmed beard stretched around a wide smile. On his head, a pointed metal helmet resembled a football with a circular brim. His legs in black stockings were shapely beneath the billow of yellow satin knickers.

Amanda sat in the backseat, staring speechless with fatigued resignation—the driver seemed to be a postcard come to life: somebody to take her to some foul-smelling fountain for healing. After all this time.

They passed between the two lions, each with one cement paw resting majestically on a little ball. Amanda remembered eating at a restaurant near the Bridge of Lions, being anxious for tall boats to come through so she could watch the bridge draw. And when it did open, how her collar had rubbed against a badly sunburned neck.

"Rain," the driver said, turning around to smile at Amanda as he flipped on the windshield wipers. By the time they pulled up in front of The Sandpiper, a steady downpour had begun. The driver honked his horn, opened the window, yelled for someone named Hector, then turned back to her: "Would you like to stay somewhere else? I know a nice motel around the—"

"No. This will be fine," Amanda said. Though she felt sick at the thought of actually sleeping in the place. Had it always looked like that? It was basically the same wood and stucco structure on the corner of the boardwalk that she remembered, but the building seemed to be eroding back into the Atlantic.

"Hector!" he yelled again. Some curtains hung outside screenless windows like wet flags on a pole. A small boy appeared in the large, open doorway of the hotel. The boy laughed, pointing at the driver who was leaning back from the window, trying not to get wet. The driver held up a single dollar bill, motioning for the boy to come. But the boy shook his head no, holding up three fingers. The driver acquiesced.

Hector ran to the car, still giggling. He brought in the suitcases—one obviously too heavy for him—while Amanda tried to get her chair out of the cab. The boy did not want to touch the wheelchair, saying, "I don't like sick people." The driver pretended to cuff him on the head, then quickly gave him another dollar. "Your father teaches you no manners. Help the lady, Hector—I'm in a hurry." And so the little boy struggled to unfold the wheelchair. Not wanting to cause more of a scene, Amanda let him push her into the lobby where vinyl-covered furniture surrounded a black-and-white television set. An old man sat watching, his walker beside him. His presence comforted her. Maybe The Sandpiper had become more like a retirement center than the crack house she feared it might be.

The boy stared at her with deep brown eyes, not saying a word. She guessed the man checking her in was Hector's father. He handed her the key with indifference. The old man on the sofa waved as she rolled past. Hector strained to manage the large brown suitcase and shopping bag full of books. Amanda placed the other bag on her lap, and they slowly made their way to the elevator.

She felt Hector's eyes stealing glances at her legs. She regretted wearing shorts. Around Cecilia, she had forgotten to be self-conscious about them. *Atrophied* was the term, though she preferred *thin*. Amanda wished she could spare the boy the discomfort he felt in looking at her, wished she could spare herself discomfort in general.

Her room smelled of old sex. She imagined a plaque boasting Site of the Oldest Fuck. Hector put the suitcase down, looking at the books wrapped in plastic bags. He looked up at Amanda, producing a cellophane bag from his pants pocket. "To warm you up, heh? Cheap, thirty-five."

"Listen, little boy."

"Don't call me that, bitch."

"I'm not retarded, OK? Thirty-five for two joints is criminal. You're a disgrace to the business."

"You sell for The Boatman?"

"No. I teach English. See, I put books in plastic bags so they don't get wet."

He looked curiously into the bag. "Read me a story then."

"Maybe later, Hector," she said, deciding she was going to get along with him after all.

"Hey, I just brought you in from the rain. I didn't say maybe later, did I?"

"OK. OK. What do you like to read?"

"Something with sex!"

"How old are you?"

"Ten, why?"

She didn't like him, after all. She unwrapped Yeats' *The Tower,* opened it, and began to read "The Mermaid." Instantly she regretted her choice. A mermaid pulls a little boy under the water to be her lover. She forgets that he cannot breathe, and so he drowns. Drowning a lover Amanda could freely discuss. But the circumstances of the poem now seemed horribly improper—and how was she going to explain the events to Hector? She thought of saying that it was a little girl mermaid that killed the little boy, but that did not seem a very good option either.

Amanda searched the brown water stains on the ceiling for solace. There was none to be found. "Well?" she asked.

"I've heard that one before."

"Yeats, you read Yeats in the fifth grade?"

"My grandfather fished. He told me about mermaids."

"Did he tell you how dangerous they are? That you should never try to touch one?"

The boy nodded. "Except for once a year when she needs the breath of a human," he added.

"My aunt told me that same story. She was a fisherman, too."

"No way! Old ladies don't get paid to fish. My grandfather sold fish to the Santa Maria Restaurant next to the Bridge of Lions." Hector walked to the window, looking out along the boardwalk. "My grandfather died."

"I'm sorry," she said. Hector was quiet then. He was an odd kid. Then he turned to her and said, "Who would want a mermaid? There's no place to stick it." He laughed a little boy laugh. A car horn blew. Someone older, not the cabbie or his father, called his name.

He bolted for the door. Then turned quickly back. "Do you need some food?"

So he wasn't all bad. Amanda decided she could trust him, despite or because of his contradictions. She handed him fifteen dollars, asked for a grouper sandwich, something to drink, and something to take the stench away. *Qué?* he asked. "Something for the smell," she said, pinching her nose with her fingers. He put both hands to his face, hiding his laughter.

She rolled to the window to see Hector getting into a beat-up old car. Already, she hoped he would be safe. Through the grey sheet of rain, the end of the massive pier was hidden from her view. And staring out the window, the wooden pier seemed merely what it was, a place to stand while fishing. No more, no less, no allegorical anything. The whole trip seemed like a gross misjudgment of need, much like her entire life at that moment.

It was her therapist's fault, asking Amanda what loss meant to her. What does it mean to anybody? Amanda had answered. Living through it was a complete pain. Still, the question had started something for Amanda.

She looked around the hotel room, wishing Cecilia was there, glad in a way that she wasn't. The water stains and the worn-out smell, maybe it was best to be alone for such self-rancor. Still, being alone there seemed like a step in some direction other than the backward one that staying home in Louisville would have been.

Just what was their problem? *The* question of the year, thought Amanda. They had met in their final year of graduate school, and in the seven years since then they had moved to just as many cities. There was no single incident, no specific fight. When together, they laughed easily, and didn't that say a lot for two basically serious people with a normal propensity for depression? And yet, for all the outward signs of content-ment between them, Cecilia seemed to be raging with equal mixes of bore-dom and discontent, hounding jobs with opera companies in bigger cities from their first day in Kentucky.

As far as sex went, Cecilia claimed that it, too, was boring—a re-minder, she said, of how peculiar sex really was if you thought about it much. Then Amanda would add that sex wasn't meant to be thought about, that it was like music, appealing to the mind in places language could never reach. To which Cecilia replied, "We've become too much like sisters to be good lovers anymore."

Amanda pondered this predicament as a sort of acquired incest, lead-ing to an irreconcilable numbness. In fact, she was more than ready to believe their relationship was decaying for a simple old-fashioned reason: a new girlfriend. A scenario that wasn't hard for Amanda to imagine, in fact she did imagine it. All sorts of women—composers, dancers, the woman who cleaned the hall late at night—any one of them eternally interesting and more capable of sweeping Cecilia off her feet.

So Amanda was simply boring. Cecilia touched her now with the distance of some tired old doctor. Gone were the sweaty explorations of how Amanda could best feel pleasure. And though Amanda knew it was dangerous to think of herself as too difficult to love, that those were the thoughts she would later pay sixty an hour to hold at bay, the dam was leaking. Besides, she wasn't difficult; it just took time. And needing time shouldn't be so awful. Cecilia was the difficult one. "Forget it," Amanda said aloud before deciding to go find a phone. Cecilia would want to be sure she was safe, though safe was anything but what Amanda felt.

Cecilia wasn't home. Amanda left a message that everything was fine. There was no one in the lobby. She hesitated to even think how the place stayed in business. Outside, the steady rain sealed the heat within the building. She rolled to the end of the covered porch to stare at the water, the pier, her past, whatever was available to think about besides what to do after vacation.

When the rain let up, she could see the end of the pier. The night of her accident, her father had been out there fishing. She had finally convinced her mother to buy her a sailor's cap from one of the gift shops. Amanda was so excited for her father to see it, she ran ahead to show him.

Sometimes Amanda was certain she could remember that last quarter mile in perfect detail. Dodging the strollers, then turning onto the wooden pier, the slight rise up from the seawall, the canopy of fishing rods arching backward with the weight of saltwater sinkers, bits of shrimp leering in front of her. A woman she called Sea Hag had just caught another catfish. She slung it down against the pier, stepped quickly on its tail. "Don't touch the son of a bitch," she said to her dog. As Amanda ran, her only worry was that the hat would blow off or be snagged by one of the casting hooks, so she kept her head up. She could still picture the shapes, mostly of men, at the end of the pier, that clump she was running toward. Then, the people and the pier with its lights were completely gone, replaced by the greenish-black of the approaching waves.

The wind shifted, causing Amanda to get wet despite the awning. A familiar vibration began in her throat, the trembling of a seam in a solitary wall. It was as if she had descended through a trapdoor into a room filled with past tense images of love—a stuffed panda bear; the sailor's cap; the tiny, muscled legs of an eight-year-old girl running to see her father; and now, Cecilia. And if she tried to touch them, her hand would merely pass through air, reminding her the room was full of loss, not of the *things* she had lost.

Amanda spent the rest of the day in her room, reading and taking notes that would eventually have to become coherent handouts for her students. Hector had not returned. The rain stopped around eight, and she decided to go out to find something to eat. Just then, there was a timid knock at the door.

Hector shoved a McDonald's bag at her, then backed away, apologizing because he had forgotten something for the smell. Tomorrow, he promised.

"Hector," she called after him, but he was gone.

She stared at the bottle inside the white bag. Pepe Lopez grinned back at her. She set the bottle down on the table, turning the label toward the wall. She did not like pictures of strange faces. As a child, a collection of masks in the children's encyclopedia frightened her. That volume had the masks of comedy and tragedy on its cover, and she always kept it face down. Amanda quickly scanned the walls for pictures of faces, but even the mirror was too high for her to see into. She poured herself a little of the tequila, feeling slightly afraid of how things were shaping up: herself alone, on the verge of leaving a woman she still loved, trying to answer what that loss would mean to her. And now her only company was Pepe Lopez. Not a good sign. She poured herself another shot.

Beneath the window she could see Hector trying to jump the curb on his skateboard. Over and over again, it never stayed beneath his feet when he went into the air. Amanda was tired of reading Yeats' autobiography. He was intrigued by masks, not frightened like Amanda. She thought of a passage, something about love, how it must wear a mask, or was it that love creates the mask?

With many of his entries, she felt a breath away from comprehension, like music or sex, something felt before being understood. But a mask meant only deception to her. Maybe to Yeats the mask was a way to hide parts of yourself, a way of keeping separate, insulated, and whole. But he also said we choose masks for our lovers, not seeing their "daily self."

She rolled to the sink, then lifted herself until she could lean her mouth close enough to the tap for a drink. There were no glasses in the room. The strong taste of sulfur caused her to spit the water out.

"We are all products of each other's imagination," Amanda said aloud. She smiled, giving in to that unique freedom that hotel rooms allow. Amanda popped her wheelchair up so that the back of the chair leaned against the bed, her hands folded casually behind her head.

Celebrating division, wearing masks, maybe it was the opposite of the principle that led people who live alone to resemble their dog or cat over the years.

Amanda leaned forward, and the small front wheels crashed against the floor. She ventured a bite of the tepid fish sandwich, washing it down with the clear liquid. Bland and sweet bitterness mingled together in her mouth, and suddenly she wished she was in some nice restaurant with Cecilia. Cecilia wearing the mask of a new lover, or maybe herself doing so.

After bashing her way into and out of the narrow bathroom door, Amanda lifted herself onto the bed, anxious for the easy transport of sleep. In the amusement park, an out-of-tune calliope began to play. Somewhere a bottle broke against the street.

The next morning Amanda awoke to a faint knock at the door. She waited for it to go away. When it didn't, she grabbed a shirt and got into her wheelchair, placing a blanket old-invalid style over her legs. Hector greeted her with yet another McDonald's bag. He smiled, handing her the bag. "Stinks," he said. "Mr. Leon will help with the stink. I've told him about you."

"Who's he, some distant relative of Ponce de León?" Amanda was taking slow sips of the coffee. Pepe had left a haze on her thoughts and tongue.

"Something like that. He owns the new RV park."

A horn blew, and Hector jumped up. "I'll be back. Mr. Leon says to take you swimming."

Amanda dealt with the bathroom again. The sink was already beginning to pull away from the wall.

After leaving another message for Cecilia at her friend's home in Santa Fe, Amanda returned to her room to read. The old man downstairs said it had been sunny that morning, too bad she missed it. Not being able to talk with Cecilia reminded her of how kids used to describe the misery of summer camp to her. Though she herself never went to summer camp, she did know the feeling of being away from her parents while in rehab centers and hospitals. She hated those memories most of all.

Amanda thought pain must be the heaviest part of memory, causing it to fall to the bottom of the mind, and sometimes, when great enough, the pit was bottomless.

When it was almost dark outside, Hector returned. Amanda had remained in her bathing suit in an effort to keep cool. Hector wore only faded cutoff shorts and sandals. He set a cardboard box down on the table, pulling a brass incense burner, two cones, and a small felt pouch of dust from inside.

"Is that stuff legal?"

"It's from Mr. Leon, I told you. You want to think I steal everything, don't you? This is his special most precious dust from Syria."

A sudden gust of wind blew out his first match. Hector was behaving quite seriously, and Amanda decided that Mr. Leon was the one who kept Hector from more serious trouble.

The smoke streamed upward, plumes of lavender deepening to dark blue.

"Won't this set off the smoke detector?"

"No. It needs batteries to work."

The smell was hardly one she'd call refreshing, having the tinge of almonds and sulfur. But stronger than any smell was the odd sense she had that the smoke was dimming the room, the hotel, the amusement park, the rain, her very thoughts, into a profound silence. A quiet that was so beautiful Amanda began to smile, almost to the point of laughing, but not laughing because of the sound that would make.

Hector remained seated on the floor, pulling one particular fray from his cutoffs over and over, the way some men stroke the same bit of hair in their beards. Looking at Hector, Amanda saw him then as a boy-man— alchemist, bellhop, small-time dealer. A public servant of sorts.

After a while, which may have been minutes or hours, Amanda could not tell, the boy-man looked up to her, saying, "It burns for a long time. We can go swimming now." And so they left the room.

The night was warm, the boardwalk empty. More than a few stars punctuated the sky. She realized then that it could be very late, maybe even close to morning.

About a half mile from the hotel there was a break in the seawall. Sea oats continued on the other side of a sandy ramp down to the beach. Hector helped Amanda as she backed the chair over the steep curb into the sand.

Once on the beach, the chair became impossible for her to push, and even with Hector's help, the small front tires were partly buried in the loose sand above the tide line. The lights from the boardwalk and a small quarter moon allowed them to see a short distance around themselves. At regular intervals, a sweep of light from the nearby lighthouse illuminated the crests of low tide's small breakers and the quick outline of the pier. Small shells crunched beneath her tires and his sandals.

"What do I do?" he asked, his feet momentarily in water as a wave ran up the sand to greet them. The lighthouse beam flashed like night lightning across the sky, and in it, Hector looked rather scared.

"Push me a little ways into the water, then make sure there are no sharp things in front of the chair. I'll lean forward and put my arms out to catch myself." As she fell forward, she knew it was a jarring sight, even if intentional.

Normally, Amanda worried about scraping her legs, but not now. Hector performed handstands, body surfing, and she, too, tried to do a flip, though it was quite unsuccessful. A wave broke over their heads, and they shrieked with laughter.

The breakers began coming more frequently, and it became hard for her to keep from washing back against the sand.

"Out here—come out here!" Hector called, waving his arm. She followed, losing sight of him when the waves swelled. She swam toward the child's voice, but even in the sweep of light, she could not see him. "Out here," she heard him call, and she continued swimming. She wasn't frightened. She was warm, her arms strong, and the voice, not really Hector's anymore, was pleasant, almost womanly.

She looked back; the lights from the boardwalk had become like stars, small dots against the black.

Then she heard a different sound, that of a woman practicing her scales. The sound of the notes urged her further out, until Amanda saw that she was beyond even the warning light on the end of the pier. Her hand brushed something solid, and she became suddenly afraid, but she saw nothing besides water. "Hector," she called. There was no answer. Only the woman's voice practicing her scales. Amanda turned, trying to locate the source, until she was moving in a frenzied, useless circle. As her arms became heavy and burned with fatigue, a thin hand grasped her own and began pulling Amanda until her back felt sand and shells against it.

At first, she was too scared to open her eyes. But when lips brushed her face, neck, breasts, descending further into the vagueness, she looked to see the glitter of the woman's silvery tail arching up and down in the water. Amanda wanted to see her face, to run her hand into her hair with its tangles of phosphorous plankton. But the woman held Amanda's arms by her side. The wet satin of scales moved onto Amanda's belly, rising up slow and precise. Then just before the woman's lips touched Amanda's, her face became the mask of tragedy from her childhood encyclopedia. And then she became Cecilia, smiling, placing her mouth over Amanda's, taking in a breath that reached to the very depth of all of Amanda's memories. And only in that brief moment did the woman allow Amanda to touch her, to lick the crusted bits of salt and algae from the corner of her mouth.

Amanda looked again to see her own face looking back and reached to touch her own, yet unfamiliar cheek. The woman pushed Amanda's hand away and began inching backward. *O rendetemi la spème, o lasciatemi morire,* she sang. Return to me my hope, or let me die. Then the woman wearing Amanda's face slipped back into the sea.

Through her tears Amanda saw the first streaks of orange straining into the eastern sky. She was safe, she was safe, she told herself over and over. Sitting up, she could see her chair several yards away. Plankton and bits of shell lined the folds of her bathing suit. And though she knew she must move as quickly as possible, part of her wanted only to lie there at the water's edge, to enjoy the incredible weight of her fatigue. But she had to go and tell someone about Hector.

She began her awkward moves toward her chair.

"Hey, over there, hey!" Hector's voice called. She turned to see the boy running, stopping briefly now and then to make sure a man was following him. Hector threw his arms around her, and she held him close, both of them wild with the smiles of relief, of knowing they had each survived. "Mr. Leon, she's OK, she's OK." Only then did she fully take in the man standing there. The man in full Castilian dress with the unmistakable legs in black stockings and buckle shoes who had picked her up at the airport.

That afternoon, Mr. Leon brought various salves from his special family collection and applied them to the cuts on her legs. She thanked him, and he smiled a wide smile before bustling out the door for a postcard shoot at the Castillo de San Marcos.

Soon, Hector burst through the door with a bag of food, this time a real grouper sandwich and fresh iced tea. For himself, expired apple pies from his friend at McDonald's. They sat together, eating in silence.

When they had finished, Amanda began putting her clothes into her suitcase.

"You're leaving, aren't you?" the boy asked.

Amanda was surprised at how hard it was to tell him yes.

"You paid for four days."

"But I've been here for years."

"*Qué?*"

Outside the hotel, waiting for the cab, Amanda sat while Hector practiced jumping the curb on his skateboard. When Mr. Leon pulled up, Hector handed her a present: the brass censer.

Amanda felt a tingling sensation in her right leg, and a swelling in her throat that was almost painful. She reached into her shopping bag, feeling for her copy of *The Tower*. She held the book for a final moment, then gave it away.

On the plane she cried a little, hoping Mr. Leon would look out for Hector as he had looked out for her in some unexplainable way. And when the flight attendants came through the cabin removing cups and trays, she thought about crazy things like trying to adopt the child, though she knew they would not exchange so much as a few lines on a postcard.

To Be Able

Billie Barbara Masten

I go out on a sunny day
It seemed dark
I felt blind

My children said
You don't answer what we ask
You answer
What you think we are saying
I felt deaf

I wanted to scream
But I had no mouth
Where are my songs?
Where are my poems?

I didn't like being a woman
Disconnected from my sexuality
Dismembered from my body
It seemed like men
Had all the power

I read about a woman
Small in stature
Lifting a car off her trapped baby
I wanted some of that

I go to the dictionary
And look up power
I find: To be able
I now know
I wasn't owning my power
My abilities

For S

Brenda Crank

You capture me in wings of verbal flight
And tangle me in webbing, glitter spun
Of words, their fibers incandescent light;
A night of fancied frenzy is begun.
How lyrical your voice, how bright the tone;
Your woven words of honey, tongue caressed,
Vibrations felt in sinew and in bone,
They lay like gentle hands upon my breasts.
Can something so impassioned last for long,
These trips of pleasure, once and now adored,
Or will these flights of fancy become song
That played too often leaves us spent and bored?
    Still, every time you touch me, it occurs;
    I come with you, and thirsty, drink your words.

Examining the Heat Exchange over a Mug of Tea

Terry Blackhawk

Soon you will reenter
this room. You will be showered,
shaved, zipped. But for now

a fractal warmth fills
my porcelain cup, fills my touch,
my skin's minutest whorls.

Reddening capillaries
activate god knows what
goddess within:

my sweet depths
where you lose yourself—
our gasps, the glow

of your skin against mine.
Where do we go then
only to return, dazed,

mussed, and set dreamily
musing, so permeable
to light passing through

these reversible blinds
I can barely reassemble myself
to sit here, to hold, trace,

infer with my pattern of prints
this patterned, heat-bearing
wall? Oh, soft, most flexible pads

enabling me to be known
and to know: radiance—
from a mug of tea!—

and the way blood carries
messages, crosses
pulse points, oxygenates itself

so that even at my fingertips
I sense my transpiring
breath, but feel no sweat, nothing

remarkable, just everyday touch,
I/you, the warmth only our bodies
can teach us, this throbbing

reaching out, this hunger
not to be alone in our
unremarkable hearts.

The Naked Truth

S. Minanel

They say our appearance really counts
that doesn't seem quite fair—
if by wearing silk, my value mounts
what happens when I'm bare?

Plastic Surgery

Mindy Kronenberg

Something about it smacks of Play-Doh
in a child's hands, the pulling
and stretching of putty into a web.
Then there is the knife itself, skating
a silent line of blood along the skin,
dividing the body from all it holds.

Can years be torn from the flesh like
the ragged hem off a skirt? The generous folds
under the chin, the pouches cushioning
the eyes like velvet pillows under
precious stones, do these deserve hating?
The etchings we were born to wear

are like maps that lead us back home. Who goes
across the continent to leave the familiar
face or voice, and finds in their own
mirror the indelible blueprint?
The surgeon's skillful lance cuts deeply
into age, failure, hurt, but leaves

the soft, malleable self intact.
Creeping along the seams of one's life is
a child clinging to what it knows,
the same small ghost of our past
who travels quietly within
and trembles at the glint of impermanence.

The Nest

Sandra Redding

"We ought to hold on to what we're given," I say. My son laughs, raises his left eyebrow as if he knows what I'm up to. I pour him another glass of iced tea, then pass the plate of deviled egg sandwiches his way. "You should have kept your tonsils," I chastise.

"They were yanked out over twenty years ago. I've never missed them." When Buddy picks up a slice of lemon, squirting some in his tea, a citrus smell neutralizes the stink of cooked eggs, freshens the kitchen.

"Your daddy and me argued against the surgery. You were so young; we didn't see the need, but the doctor kept insisting."

"Mama, I had throat infections. Don't you remember?"

"You would've probably outgrown the sickness. If I had it to do over—"

Buddy pats my arm indulgently, as if he thinks I'm not quite right in the head. I back away. "You clear your throat a lot. Maybe you wouldn't if you still had tonsils."

"I'm fine, Mama." He speaks sharply, but later his voice softens, becomes almost velvety with concern. "How about you? *You* OK?"

I look around. Visible bite marks, those made by Buddy at age three, mar the end of the maple table where we sit. In the corner, my ancient refrigerator shakes, rattles, and rolls as if protesting all the cantaloupes, cucumbers, and fresh-picked corn crammed inside. "Well," I confess, nodding toward the empty canning jars lined up on the kitchen counter, "I haven't felt like putting up beans and tomatoes lately."

"What is it?"

"Women's problems."

Buddy blushes. He's always been tender that way. His red face makes me feel awkward. "No use being embarrassed," I tell him. "You're nearly thirty, and married. Surely Lou Anne's mentioned such things."

When my son's eyes meet mine, I notice he still looks much the way he did as a boy: sandy hair, a swarm of freckles flying across his nose, though they've paled some, not quite so noticeable. I used to worry that his ears were too big, but now they balance his broad face, and his fingernails are always clean. He works as an accountant; he can't afford boyhood smudges.

Finishing his sandwich, he intertwines his fingers, waits until I serve the banana pudding. On his right hand he wears his college ring, the stone deep blue, winking in the sunlight that beams through the window. A wide wedding band marks the ring finger of his left hand. Above, circling his wrist, is a Rolex. Though he hasn't mentioned it, I suspect the thing's real, not the fake kind.

"Tell me, Mama," he says, "what is this illness? What can I do to help?"

I grin. "Put your hand on my head and shout 'Heal!'"

Buddy hee-haws. I laugh too. But then, God bless him, he actually does it, his fingers pushing hard into my scalp, saying *Heal* in the most reverent tone, just as if that might make a difference.

"This doctor I've been going to." I start.

"The *woman* doctor?"

"Well, anyway, she says my womb's got to go. She says it's such an ugly thing, big, out of shape. Can you imagine, badmouthing a person's insides like that?"

Buddy stares at the floor. "Is it cancer?"

"Of course not. That's the problem, don't you see? In her words, my uterus has lost its function, so why leave it there. According to her 'There's a potential for future problems.'"

"There must be something."

"Fibroids," I tell him. "Harmless tumors that usually begin to shrink a year or so after *the change*."

Buddy blushes again.

"She's just eager," I say. "Probably hasn't had too many opportunities to cut on people."

"You told me you liked her."

"Well, as doctors go, I suppose she's all right. At least before she started this business about surgery."

"Maybe she's right."

"Dr. Vyas thinks so."

"Two doctors have advised this, Mama?"

"He's still in his twenties."

"If two say it—"

"There's more than one fool in the world."

My son shakes his head.

As we eat our banana pudding from blue-speckled plates, light seeps through the window again, holding us in a soft glow. Buddy finishes the last of the iced tea. "Would you like me to look into it for you?" he wants to know.

"Yes," I deadpan. "Call a meeting of all your accountant friends, and ask them what I should do. Have them put together some numbers, and get back to me with the odds."

Buddy laughs. "Damn, Mama, you just won't do."

Sitting there, licking my spoon, I think back to the last Christmas before Buddy's daddy died. The tree we had that year, a fresh balsam, was decorated just the same as the year before and the year before that. Always practically the same. A silver peace symbol on the top and twinkle lights: red, green, yellow, white.

"Remember," I ask my son, "the bluebird's nest that we always placed on the Christmas tree?"

"I found the thing beneath the oak tree. The one that still grows in the side yard."

"You brought it inside, begging me to put it up in the oak again so the mama bird would lay more eggs."

"You claimed she wouldn't."

"You cried, Buddy, 'cause it meant something to you. So although the thing was moldy and filled with bird poop, I fastened it to the Christmas tree and every year after that, even after the fool thing fell apart."

My son reaches for my hand, rubs his finger back and forth over the blue vein that snakes beneath the skin. "We can't always hold on to a thing," he tells me.

"But the nest looked right up there, don't you think?" I ask him. "A reminder of the mama bird and the baby birds."

Buddy gets up, takes his glass to the sink, rinses it out, places it in the dishwasher. When he comes back, he rubs my shoulder. "Well, Mama, what will you decide?"

I think long and hard before speaking. "How am I to know what's right?"

His blue eyes seek mine. "Is it worth taking chances?"

"If we're to believe those white coats, practically everything we do is risky."

My son grins. After glancing at his Rolex, he bends, kisses me on the cheek. "I've got to get back to the office."

He puts on his coat. Blue-and-white striped, not a wrinkle. From his pocket he takes a roll of breath mints. He offers them to me. I take one and he takes one, and soon we both smell minty as juleps. "Well," I say as I walk with him toward the door, "I suppose I will."

"Will what?"

"Be cut on."

My son takes both my hands. "You sure? You can still get another opinion. As many as you want, Mama."

"They're all in cahoots. It'd be the same."

"When?"

"The sooner, the better, I suppose."

He hugs me. "Whatever time you decide, I'll be with you. You do know that, don't you?"

I pat his back. Then I get this idea, clear as window glass, just the way I want it to turn out. If the thing's got to be done, then it'll be done proper.

"Now, Mama, what're you up to?" Buddy asks when he sees me smile. He's like that, zooming in on my mischievousness even before it's fully bloomed.

"We'll plant it in the yard," I tell him plainly.

Buddy appears puzzled. "Plant what?"

I leave time for what I've said to sink in. It takes a while.

Finally he strides resolutely back to the kitchen table, yanks the chair out, sits down. "Now, Mama," he speaks in his clipped accountant tone, the voice he uses when discussing business. He spreads his fingers out as if he intends to count them. "Let me get this straight. What exactly will you be planting?"

I pause, waiting for him to calm down before I answer. "My insides," I finally say. "All they cut out."

He spreads his fingers over his face, peeps at me through them. "Lord help."

I say nothing. He shakes his head. "You do get such *strange* notions. Even stranger now than when Daddy was alive."

"The hospital will let me have my uterus, won't they, Buddy?"

"I suppose so."

"Then I intend to see the thing put in the ground, with or without your help."

He acts peevish. "I didn't say I wouldn't help."

"The hydrangea in the side yard's been looking puny; some of the leaves have yellowed. We'll plant it there. Maybe it'll perk up."

Buddy laughs.

I touch his sweet face.

"Well, Mama," he asks, "exactly how elaborate will this burial be? I hope you aren't expecting a eulogy or song from me?"

I look at him steady, examine my own reflection in his clear blue eyes. "No need to plan anything fancy," I answer. "A short prayer will suit just fine."

This Insane Notion, She Says

Grace Butcher

A baby at sixty. The eggs in there like tiny pearls. The fishy sperm swimming their best till they hit the road block and the long tunnel closed off; they die in darkness.

The uterus, ageless, suddenly waiting again. That unlit room where everything happened so long ago. But she dreams of it, youth still hovering like an aura she knows he sees.

She is mysterious to him: surely she could do this one most simple thing. She wills herself untied. He has freed her from every curse ever laid upon her, kissed her awake after such a long sleep, surely she could make this simple thing happen, let just one of those million swimmers slip past that barricade.

Think how the egg would glow with joy, feeling itself finally useful. Think how the uterus would turn on all its black lights, how they would shine into all its round corners, shine onto this fish, this pearl, this watery joining, lapped by dark waves.

She doesn't think beyond this scene; no dream roads lead out from it. What emergence into daylight would mean, she has no idea.

Love, she says. It makes you crazy. Most of her friends agree though a few catch her smiling. They know she is capable of just about anything.

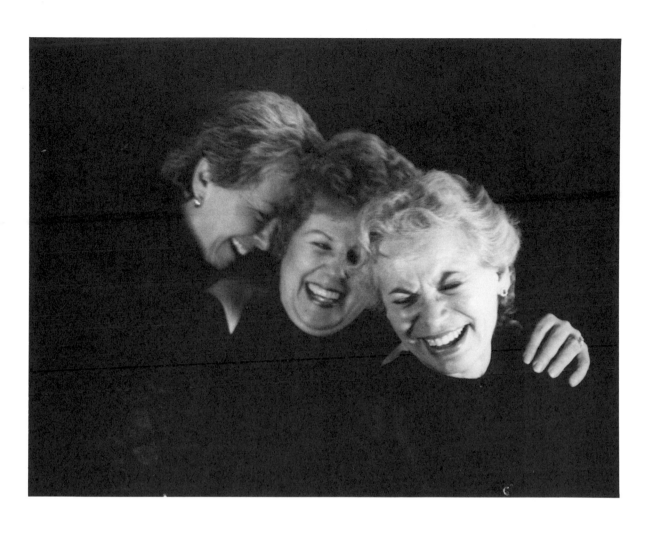

Take My Body

Elizabeth Weber

I bequeath my left shinbone
to my daughter to make out
of it all that can be made:
a white clasp for her hair, buttons

for a favorite sweater,
a necklace with the various
faces of the moon so beauty
will follow her as she followed

me. Let her form a pen
from my right forearm bone, detailed
with all the first words: mama,
papa, no, why, don't, bye-bye. Out of

my other arm let her make
a letter opener carved with
snakes and tigers. As she
opens letters from her lovers, let

her think of waking to her own
wilderness and danger.
Out of my breast bone let her
carve a knife to use when

danger comes. Out of my pelvic
bone, the ocean we come from
and then finally die into,
daughter, like a shell put it

to your ear and listen
to the waves rock you, listen
for the voices of those beyond
you, before you, those who fed you,

held, cleaned, set you on your feet
and let you go to stumble
and fall. The skull is nothing:
give it to the cat to play with.

Crone Drives through Spring

Claudia Van Gerven

She can hardly bear to look
out the window:
earth seems to break
loose, fidgets, squirms, restless spasms
of green, and the sky
a whirligig of birds. She cannot keep
the car on the road: it wants
to canter across fields abandoned
to the wanton purple of
tiny nameless flowers. The precision of
snow unbuttons itself
like a girl's blouse, but she is too old
to come spilling out, unlatching
the seat belts, freeing the Toyota.
What would they make of
this aging runner, white hair streaming
down her stooped back, slack
thighs vaulting irregularly
down the astonished creek bank?
What could she be but
an embarrassment
to traffic laws?
to city building codes?

Combustion

Susan Carol Hauser

I took a sauna once, long ago, in a shed on the shore of a northern lake. I leaned back, closed my eyes, and let the heat come over me. My heart rate picked up. My shoulders slumped. I might as well have been standing in rain, my body awash in water. I was the chicken sort and did not finally dive into the lake, but I did stand out in the night and let the air nibble me dry.

I felt good afterward, lighter and emptied, relieved of the weight of all that sweat that had been lurking inside me. I sat for a long time content to just sit, and then had a good sleep, the kind that comes when you've left one day behind and the next is still in shadow.

That was about twenty-five years ago. I've had a lot of good sleeps since then, but forgot about the beauty of a gratuitous sweat. Forgot about it until a few years ago when my personal female sauna kicked in. Hot flashes. Hormone storms. The fireworks that signal the end of fecundity. A prolonged celebration of the rite of passage that is menopause.

Back on that night of the induced sweat, my younger son Aaron declined to join us. One ladle of water on those benign looking rocks sent him and his five-year-old body fleeing into the safety of the night. He couldn't quite leave us though. He pressed his face against the rough wall and peered at us through a large crack. We could see his one eye, opened wide like a mouth.

When I have a hot flash, part of me feels like Aaron. I watch, astounded, as an invisible hand tosses water on the stones of my body, and I ignite. How can flesh not melt? Then, of necessity, I give up the watch and close my eyes and float on the water, and then the fire expends itself, and I pick up my little fan and create a breeze something like the ones that frequent northern lakes at night. Then I just sit in the quiet puddle of my flesh. If it is the middle of the night I sleep the good sleep of a person cleansed.

Of course, not all of the storms come in the privacy of my home. They come during meetings, during lunch downtown, at the grocery store, on the street corner while I am in conversation with a passerby friend. Awe strikes the company I keep, their eyes widening as a child's at the scene: my face turning red, water erupting on my brow, my glasses steamed, my arms windmills as I cast off as many layers of clothing as decorum allows while searching for a tissue to sop the water out of my eye wells.

Yes, I'm all right, I tell them. Not having a heart attack, just a hot flash, news from the body front: this woman is shedding the garment of the lunar clock. Marvel at it with her, at her luck in carrying within herself an organic sauna. Any time, any place, she may slip away for a few minutes into a wash of free-flowing sweat.

Envy her. It is making her strong, is tempering her with the fire and water contained whole within her human body.

Osteoporosis

Mary Zeppa

Morbid absorption of bony substance
to which small-boned women
are particularly prone.

For a woman's small bones
may turn brittle
and a woman's thin spine

may turn mean, may say No
to the burden her flesh makes
once the long downslide

begins. For once the skeleton
starts its good-byes, and once
the slow creaking starts,

once the hot roses flash—
belly, breasts, face—
it's the slick-with-sweat shine

of hot flesh melting down
while the battered, defiant, old heart
pumps the pound-foolish blood

toward the catch in the throat
for the quick and the dead
and the lost.

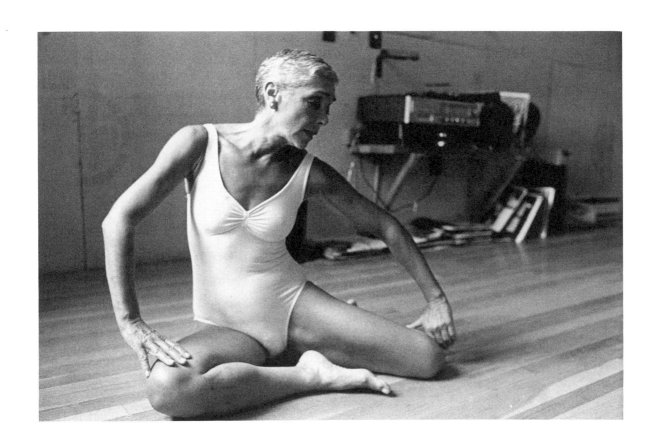

Lucy

Kathleen Patrick

If dreaming is remembering, Lucy,
how close do I come to the volcanic heat
of your world? You, the riddle
we thought we solved when your bones
were unearthed, preserving the answer
to the earliest human, the first mother
yet to be found.
Your pelvis, an open butterfly like mine,
knew childbirth, felt the cycles of the moon.
Your feet like my feet, but smaller,
your hands, my hands.
We have touched children, you and I.
The earth is still here, struggling to survive.
And when I dream of you in the deep night
my tongue speaks in guttural sounds,
asks you female questions, invites you
to sit by my fire. What is locked in the brain
of the past? What do I carry around with me still?
What do we all know?
What have we always known?

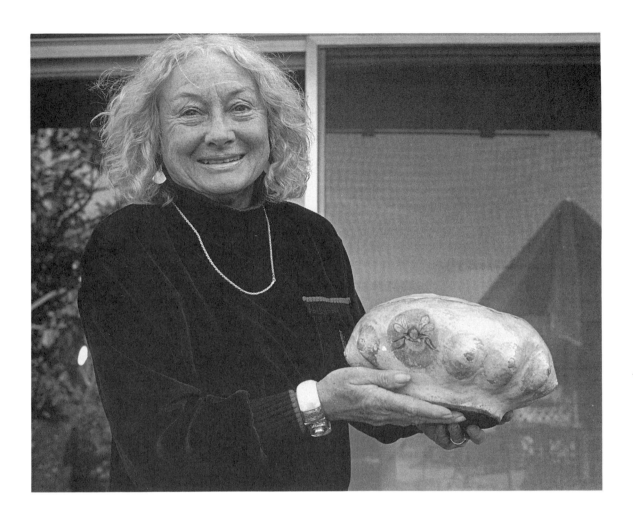

Rehabilitation

Elaine Rothman

Somewhere she had read that the ancient Egyptians believed the heart was the seat of all memory, all thought, all desire. That was why, when they removed the other internal organs while preparing a body for mummification, they left the heart in place. She had been thinking a lot about this ancient practice lately, ever since her own heart had stopped beating. It had failed for a crucial period of time, the doctors said, but medical science intervened and saved her at the last moment.

That had been seventy days ago. This morning, for some reason, she had counted the days since her heart attack, and considered the number to have a mysterious significance. Because she also remembered reading that the ancient Egyptians embalmed their dead by immersing a body for seventy days in a special, dehydrating salt bath. Natron, the salt was called. She recalled trying to find that particular reference among the files where she stored clippings, pictures, all kinds of information on long-gone civilizations. It had probably been discarded, no longer in existence, like the lives of all the ancient peoples.

"A waste of time," her father had pronounced her preoccupation with the past. "It's some kind of obsession with you, collecting all that junk. Where are we going to find the space for it all?" And every summer, when she returned from her week at her grandmother's, she would find her old *National Geographics*, the ones that she'd managed to buy at tag sales for a nickel apiece, gone. She never protested the loss of her collection, because she understood the reason for the clean sweep. Although the barns on the family farm might be immense, their dwelling was only four small rooms.

Her mother had been slightly kinder. "I wish you wouldn't buy all that smelly old stuff, dear. You never know where people have kept those books and things," she would say, adding, "When I was a girl I used to read lots of stories about long ago, too, mostly fairy tales." Her mother never failed to assure her that the real world was a far more satisfying place, especially if you worked hard at things that mattered.

Now, decades later, she still read voraciously, fascinated by stories, authentic or imagined, about people who lived centuries ago. Each fall she looked longingly at the community college catalog that arrived in the mailbox. She would linger on the first page, where introductory courses in anthropology, archaeology, and art history were listed, before tossing it out, along with the descriptions of exotic trips and catalogs for luxurious undergarments that had also come, addressed to Occupant, in the same mail.

She still saved news clippings, filing the latest among those yellowed and crumbling with age. At used book sales she had discovered old *Smithsonian* magazines to supplement copies of newly collected *National Geographics.* Stacks of pictures, periodicals, and newspapers grew to satisfying heights, only to diminish as it became apparent that there was no space for her stuff, at first in her apartment, and then in the succession of houses in which she lived.

The real world her mother had promised her turned out to be life with a husband who ran an automobile brake and muffler repair franchise, and two sons who breathed crankcase oil and could fix anything driven by a motor. She saw that somehow there was always room in the current basement, garage, or toolshed for anything metal or greasy, in working order, or with practical possibilities. Her own books on Roman togas, Dead Sea Scrolls, and the pyramids were probably frivolous anyway.

She had never lived with anyone who wasn't practical. Everything was valued according to what it could do or what it could buy. The interest that her father had called her obsession with the past, her husband and sons thought of as a harmless hobby. Not very subtly they put their heads together and encouraged another pastime of hers: sewing, quilting, different kinds of handiwork.

Remarking that she knitted great sweaters and that there was no reason she couldn't make a little money out of her skills, her husband built her a shop where she could sell yarn, spools of thread, all kinds of sewing and knitting supplies. The boys built a large trestle table where she could measure bolts of fabric. The shop was located in an outbuilding, well back from their home, at the end of a rutted lane, overlooking a pond. She saw that at last there would be plenty of space for her books and magazines, even for a battered, metal filing cabinet.

However, at this moment the yarn shop was locked, window shades drawn. The sign that her husband had tacked to the door saying, Temporarily Closed Due to Illness, had brought her dozens of get well cards, and a few handmade, whimsical stuffed animals from her regular customers.

When this cardiac rehabilitation thing was over, she might reopen her shop and find herself once again reading quietly near the corner window overlooking the pond. At the tinkle of a bell announcing the occasional customer, she would probably glance up at the rainbow of woolen spools she had displayed on ceiling-high shelves and arrange a pleasant expression on her face. She would hope she had stocked exactly what the person needed, so the customer would pick it up and leave. The best days were when no one at all drove up the rutted lane.

This morning she looked around the long, corridor-like rehabilitation room, humming and clanking with machinery. Some of the racket was absorbed, she supposed, by the water-stained acoustical tiles on the low ceiling. The walls might have been drab except for the posters, plastered haphazardly and covered with cartoon characters, Day-Glo letters, and exclamation points. Count Your Calories! Watch Your Blood Cholesterol! Take Your Medicine Regularly! Aerobic Exercise Is the Thing! Learn How to Deal with Stress! If she narrowed her eyes, the messages became indecipherable, like hieroglyphics. At the far end of the room were wheeled carts on which patients lay, ministered to by physical therapists.

Her portion of the room was where six women, herself included, worked out on various moveable contraptions. They all wore identical, tomato red T-shirts emblazoned with Cardiac Rehabilitation over flat chests, or sagging breasts, or, in one case, provocatively pointed nipples. Every face was red with exertion, sweaty with effort, and grim with purpose. All of them, even the pointy-breasted one, had pasty white thighs that jiggled.

Apart from the uniform, she had nothing in common with any of the others in her class, except for a recent heart attack and the shuddering, vibrating machines on which they perched, three times a week for twelve weeks. It wasn't very likely that anyone was considering embalming techniques, as she was, or making the time pass by imagining ancient priests working at the other end of a long, communal tomb. She knew for a fact that one woman was wondering when she would be permitted to rejoin her bowling club, and another figuring how many children she could safely monitor in her backyard swimming pool. Just before the warm-ups, a series of arm stretching, knee bending, and floor-swoops, they had told her so.

People always told her things about themselves. "You have a face with listening eyes," her husband once said. Yet she could not allow herself to exchange confidences. For instance, her husband and sons would be devastated to learn she didn't really enjoy needlework. It was just something to do, something she was good at. If she told them that, after all their hard work in providing her with the shop, they would think her ungrateful.

She much preferred reading. She had even tried balancing a book on the handlebars of one of these Exercycles, but in twelve minutes all she had been able to absorb was a page or two. Even the stereo, meant to provide pleasant background music, emitted a muffled murmur, drowned by the clank of bicycles and the thud of treadmills. Eventually the hour would pass, and an hour wasn't a lifetime after all.

She had to admit that she felt pretty good, after the initial anguish of the heart attack and the despair of the weakness that followed. There was something to be said for taking control of your own recovery. And there were no crybabies in this class. No one who wanted to tell horror stories over the scales or the blood pressure machines. Only a few superficial jokes as they all poked under their red shirts to secure the square monitoring box and three wired tabs into their strategic places.

She appreciated the kindness of one woman, the bowling club person, sharp-eyed enough to notice her ineptness with fastening those wires in their proper places. At the beginning of every session, she silently accepted the woman's help, smiling her thanks. She did not mention how intimidating she found anything mechanical, at the same time how awestruck she was by the miracles machines could accomplish.

The night before her operation, she had shared a room with a woman who expressed the frightening thoughts skimming in her own head.

"If you should die, what would you miss most?" the woman had asked her in a soft, wondering voice.

"I suppose I'd miss my books," she'd answered tentatively.

Then they began to talk of summertime because in a few weeks it would be summer. She found herself saying she'd miss the taste of wild strawberries, each one like a minuscule spoonful of jam; the sight of a snapping turtle poking his nose through the pond lilies; the explosion of light in the nighttime shrubbery as fireflies teased each other with, "Where are you?" and "Right over here!" Of course, she had stopped short of telling her roommate how she'd miss bringing her husband's hand to her lips and lightly kissing every knuckle until he turned to her in his sleep, reaching out for her mouth and then her whole body.

At first her throat had ached with the unaccustomed revelations, as if a heavy chain scraped along her gullet, dragging the words from her. Then the talk slipped from her easily. She spoke for hours, almost gratefully, until they both slept, and in the morning the woman was gone.

Never before had she shared any of her feelings with anyone for fear of being thought fanciful, or foolish. "She's got a Mona Lisa smile. She's a riddle. Reads too much about the sphinx, if you ask me." She was used to people talking about her as if she weren't there. Even people who cared about her.

Yes, the ancient Egyptians were right. The heart must be the seat of all yearning. When the sharp pain struck her left shoulder, like a spearpoint penetrating all the way to her breast, when the nausea rose in her throat so that she knelt in front of the toilet and spewed up everything in her guts, when her lungs refused to accept any air so that she felt suffocated, all yearning stopped except the desire to escape from the hurting.

Yet for a long time there was to be no escape. She had to remain awake throughout her own surgery. She was expected to lie there watching a screen on which a thin black wire snaked through her artery. She had to be alert and ready to take deep breaths or cough on demand, when all she wanted to do was to slip into oblivion. And when it was over, she hid her bruised, purplish body, tattooed by the machines that first assaulted before they rescued. For weeks she stayed clothed from neck to ankle, ashamed of her appearance and her weakness, yet never complaining, in case someone would think she was a whiner.

Now, in the seventy-first day of renewed life, she watched the sinews in her arms stretch as she pushed the handlebars of an Exercycle forward and backward at an individually prescribed speed. Hooked up to the wires under her red T-shirt, she glanced at the bright green, wavy lines alight on a screen, lines that signified her heartbeat. She recalled the array of other devices she'd encountered in the past couple of months: mechanical balloons and reamers, clamps and pressure packs, catheters, pumps, scanners, and monitors. With every rotation of the pedals, every alternating stroke of the handlebars, she reviewed the names of the incomprehensible machinery that had circumscribed her days and weeks.

At the designated time she relinquished her bike to the young woman with the firm, pointy breasts and moved over to a treadmill, her favorite exercise. Striding up a never ending hill, she shifted her weight from one leg to the other in a confident saunter, barely touching the side rails with the tips of the fingers of one hand. Why had the attack occurred in her case? There was probably no one reason, she had been told, perhaps a com-

bination of several. Just follow all those instructions on the posters plastered all around her, and it might not happen again.

The others in the class had begun to change their stations for the last
time that morning, propelled by the reminders posted on a blackboard.
She exchanged her treadmill for a stationary bike, the most monotonous
machine of all, but cooling if she pedaled fast enough to set the fan going.
The undulating lines that were her heart's measure scratched a steady
progress, and the eerie numbers flashed reassuringly low.

She let her thoughts flow back to ancient Egypt. She had once found a
most memorable picture in the endpaper of a news magazine. She hoped
it hadn't been thrown out in one of their frequent moves. If it had, it
wouldn't matter, because she knew the face in the picture as well as her
own.

It was a full-page photo of the reconstructed head of an Egyptian
woman, taken from a mummy on exhibit at the Indianapolis Children's
Museum. Wenu-hotep was the woman's name, *hotep* for "in honor of,"
Wenu for who knows what, and the two together pronounced as a whisper
and a kiss. She had repeated the name over and over because the survival
of a name, according to the ancient Egyptian belief, meant the survival of
a personality, even after death.

She could still see the woman in the photograph, breathtakingly beautiful. Her skin was smooth, the color of bittersweet chocolate. Intelligence
gleamed from her long lashed, dark eyes. Her brows were feathery, her
cheekbones broad and well defined, her lips sensuous. Her rounded, well-
shaped skull was shaved, ready for the heavy black wig that would shield
her from the brutal Egyptian sun.

When she had first studied the picture of what Wenu-hotep must have
looked like in life, she wondered about the things the Egyptian woman
left behind her: the fragrance of lotus and tamarisk, the early morning cry
of the ibis, the taste of fried honey cake, the kinds of things she and the
woman in the next hospital bed had talked about.

For three thousand years Wenu-hotep had lain in her coffin, bones
blackened and brittle, flesh fallen away to a crumble of resin and salt.
Only her linen wrappings kept the curious eyes of the living from gazing
on the indignities of death. Then, the newspaper said, a Chicago professor,
using computer-generated data, had her face recreated on a computer
screen and a photograph made of the result. Technology had taken a dry
mummified skull and returned the warmth and roundness of living flesh

to it. Machines had restored Wenu-hotep's womanhood, along with her name.

A sudden silence jarred her out of her reverie. She realized that the noise of every machine but hers had ceased. Even the stereo was quiet. She hopped off the Exercycle and joined the group of red-shirted women in a series of orchestrated, cooldown calisthenics. Next they were all expected to select a cup of juice from the tray on a nearby table, and to take a seat.

Almost oblivious to the buzz of voices around her, she sipped at her juice, waiting for her heart to slow to an acceptable rate, and thinking hard about the latest college catalog. It was the first that she had not discarded the same day it had come in the mail. If she should decide to enroll as a full-time student, there would be no point in reopening the yarn shop as a place of business. Yet it would be a shame to let the little building go to waste, when it was an ideal place for what she knew to be her real work. The whole idea was certainly worth thinking about.

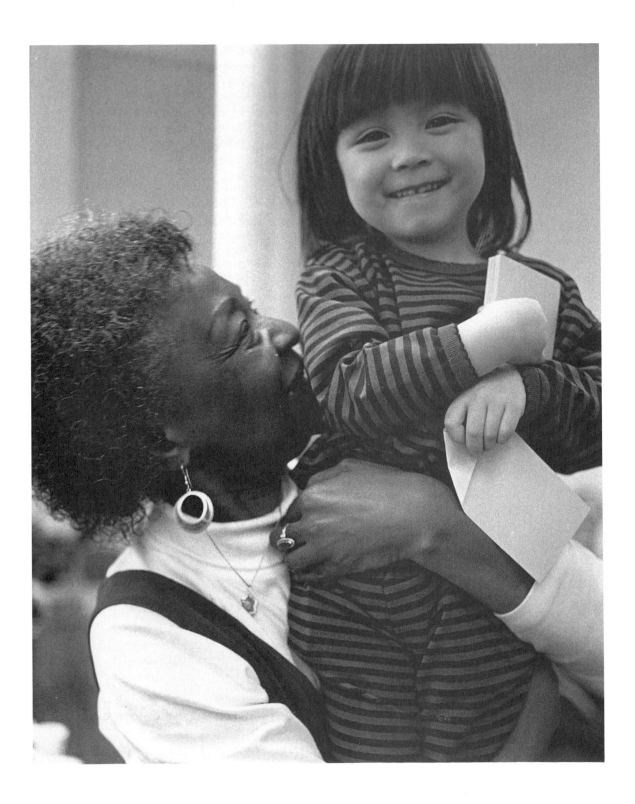

After Sixty

Marilyn Zuckerman

The sixth decade is coming to an end.
Doors have opened and shut.
The great distractions are over—
passion   children   the long indenture of marriage.
I fold them into a chest I will not take with me when I go.

Everyone says the world is flat and finite
on the other side of sixty.
That I will fall clear off the edge into darkness,
that no one will hear from me again
—or want to.

But I am ready for the knife slicing into the future,
for the quiet that explodes inside,
to join forces with the strong old woman,
to give everything away and begin again.

Now there is time to tell the story,
time to invent the new one—
to chain myself to a fence outside the missile base,
to throw my body before a truck loaded with phallic images,
to write Thou Shalt Not Kill on the hull of a Trident submarine,
to pour my own blood on the walls of the Pentagon,
to walk a thousand miles with a begging bowl in my hand.

There are places on this planet
where women past the menopause
put on tribal robes,
smoke pipes of wisdom
—fly.

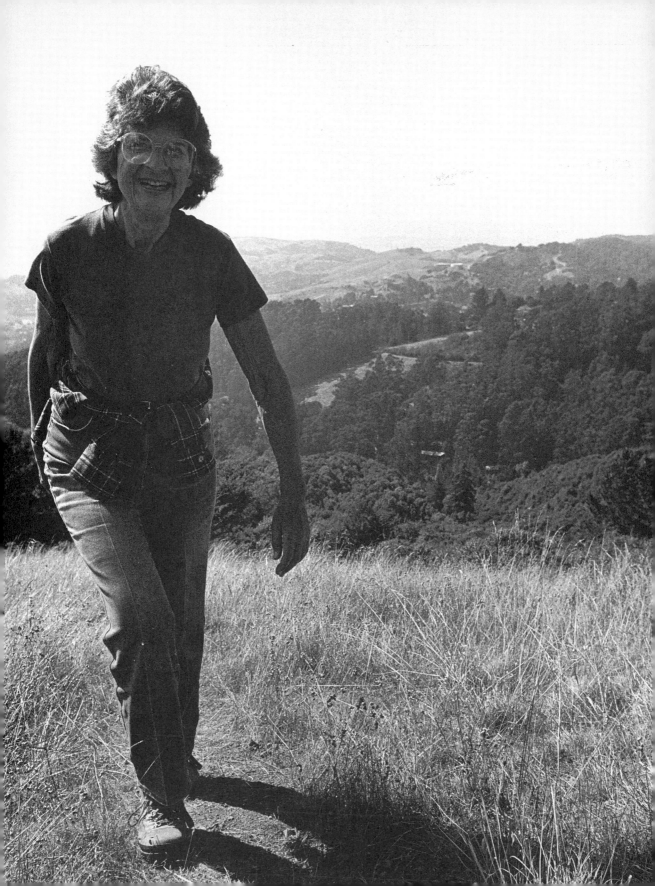

Clay

Sarah Allen

On the cusp of sleep I am simply Sarah, ageless. As I awake there is a moment like that when a lump of clay becomes centered on the potter's wheel. I feel myself spinning out from the core of self, becoming a vessel that is no longer the solid soul but a container for the soul.

Summer heat hovers just beyond the whirling blades of the ceiling fan. The sheets are tangled around bare legs, gown twisted above my hips by the night's thrashing. I kick them away and roll to the side of the water bed. When I pull the chain of the fan, the room is still. Mockingbirds sing in the oleanders. Sunlight slants through the tilted blinds sending parallel ribbons of pale light across pictures on the wall, imprisoning my children and grandchildren with transparent bars.

Glancing in the wide mirror over the dresser, I glimpse my blurred face as I choose a pair of shorts and cotton underpants. There is smug pleasure in passing over the neatly rolled bras that are only called into service on special occasions. Their straps and hooks no longer torture me. My body hosts an interesting assortment of growths and discolorations. A scattering of small moles has spread beneath my breasts, sheltering in the soft fold. Freckles have surrendered to age spots that appear across my hands and face in strange constellations. The years I spent courting the Sun God are paid for with trips to a dermatologist to make sure cancer hasn't invaded the tissues of my body.

This year I bought six shirts, loose cotton with two pockets placed for modesty. These and four pairs of shorts are my summer uniform. I no longer work in the outside world, struggling into clothes that conform to standards of current style and beauty. This freedom is a gift that pleases me anew each day.

Brushing my teeth I'm grateful for the hours spent in dentist's chairs while someone cleaned, polished, and filled. There are crowns and two teeth that are mine by virtue of someone's skill and my money, but most of them are homegrown. I notice that under my upper arm the skin and muscle have slipped into a relaxed and jiggling dance with gravity. The skin is textured like washed silk, not so much wrinkled as lightly crushed by the years.

Being nearsighted, aging has brought a little clarity to my distance vision. There is now an area some three feet away where I can see details that were hidden to me without glasses when I was younger. When I look at the sky or a blank canvas, there is a scrim of coarse netting that drifts across my vision, moving away and back again. When I first noticed it, I was frightened enough to make an appointment with my ophthalmologist. *Cataracts, glaucoma,* were words that had come into my vocabulary with my mother's later years.

"It's fairly common for nearsighted people to experience detached vitreous after fifty. For some reason it seems to bother women more than men. You're one of the lucky ones. The retina wasn't torn when the vitreous detached. It's happened in both eyes. Do you know when?"

"About two months ago I was working on some needlepoint when I thought I saw a scrap of white paper sail across the room from the corner of my eye. It was after that."

"You should have called then. If your retina had torn, you would have needed immediate surgery to save your sight. Well, that's behind you. It shouldn't happen again. Some people see the floating vitreous as a sprinkling of black pepper across their vision. There's nothing we can do. You have no signs of cataracts or glaucoma. You'll just have to live with the rest. The eye may absorb some of it, or it may move out of your central vision."

That was three years ago. It hasn't gotten better, but I adjusted to it. Amazing how the mind can register something, identify it, and then ignore it.

The shorts are size sixteen. After my four children were born, I wore a ten, comfortably. My body has stored a layer of plumpness around the middle where there was once a very small waist. I'm glad I enjoyed it while I had it. Sometimes I feel like I'm eternally four months pregnant, the stage when you become straight between chest and hips. I've spent the last ten years of my life searching for dresses that swing from the shoulders, allowing movement and a sense of freedom. Before her eyesight failed, Mother made me six dresses. We found a pattern where gathers fell from front and back yokes. These dresses were gentle on my body, graceful when I moved, and the most comfortable things I ever owned. There was one point of disagreement between us. Mother refused to put pockets in them. It was her firm belief that ladies did not put their hands in pockets. I love pockets. I wore these dresses until the fabric was as thin as tissue paper. There are only two left. One day I'll slit the side seams and put in pockets.

Dressing in the quiet apartment, I feel familiar dichotomy. The sudden panic of not having a schedule wars with the delight of a day to structure as I wish. There is time for a second cup of coffee and a few minutes on the balcony looking out over the bay for dolphins. I learn to move slowly, taking more time for small chores.

My husband buys me canvases. They are stacked against the closet door in the spare room, also my studio. He never asks when I will start one, but as they are finished, he buys another. There is an immense feeling of richness in my life.

The busy-ness of living has been reduced to an essential lump of clay, wedged and cut on the wire of sixty-one years until all the air pockets are gone. There is a dense, heaviness that, devoid of extraneous material, is only myself. I can spin it through the coming days into a form that pleases me, pulling it up into a cylinder where the clay is thin and slippery, pressing it down again, pulling it out into a wide bowl to hold all that is me.

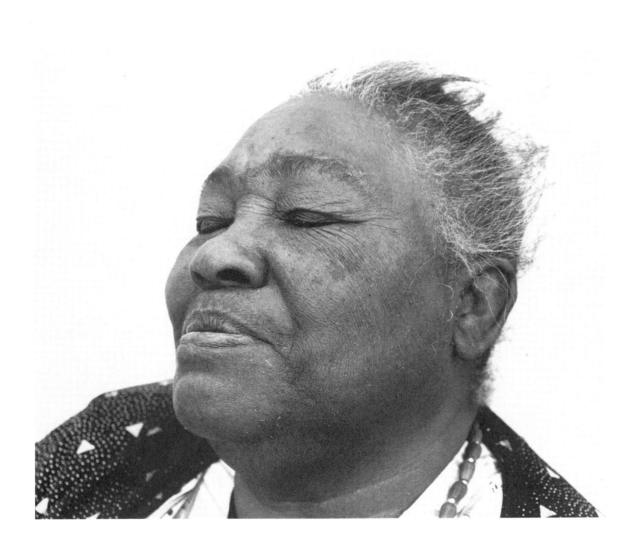

Spring Surge

Kay Loftus

My blood still answers to the hawk's wild cry,
Although my years are many, and the fine,
Clean edge of passion dulled by long disuse.

Love now is gentler. And the more diffuse
Emotion of compassion is most often mine.
Yet in me passion's remnants will not die.

In Praise

Mary Sue Koeppel

I like the sound
of old women
marching to church,
or crackling grocery bags,
or eating stewed prunes,
and sugar on tomatoes.

I like the sound
of old women
talking
loudly to old men,
softly to newborns,
gently to young marrieds,
planning lives and death.

I like the sound
of old women
snoring,
old women
clicking teeth,
old women
praying.

I like the sound
of old women
raucously in love.
I like the sound
of old women
roistering in helpless
rollicking fun.

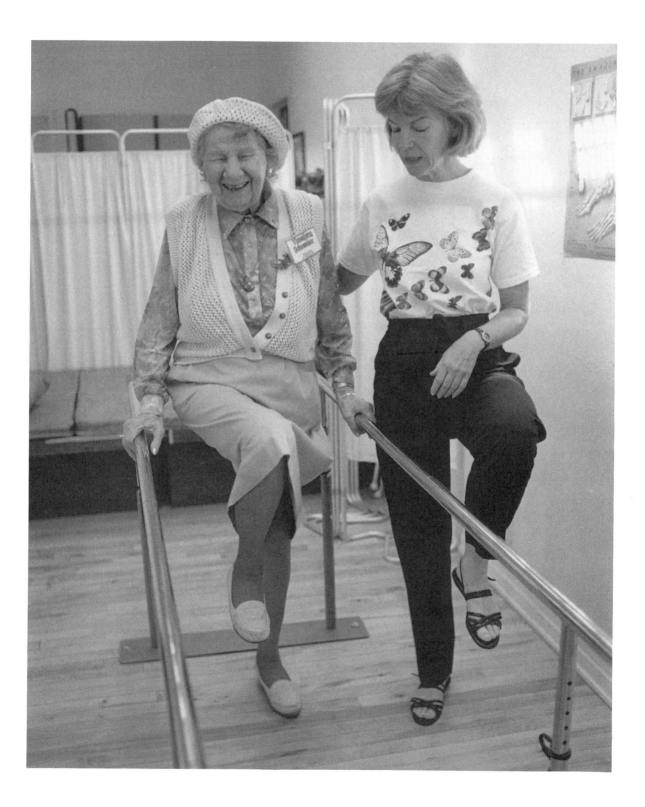

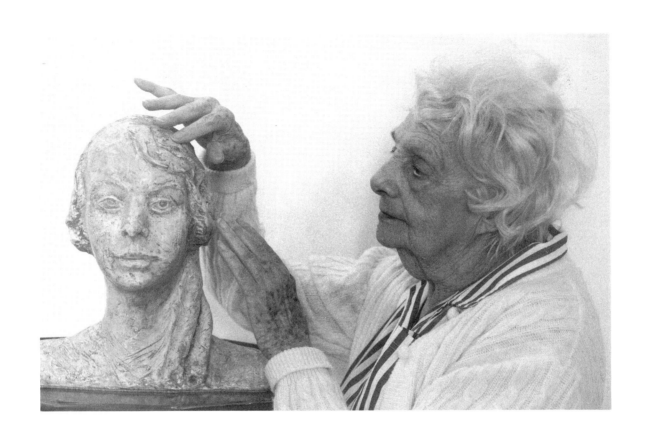

Volunteer Mourner

Marie Kennedy Robins

I like to go places. I like to flit.
I'd even to go the opening of an envelope.
But buryings are really the top of my line.
I know how to send folks off to their Maker
so He knows they're coming and opens the door.

After Elbert went upstairs, I was lonesome.
I got me a road dog with fleas and a porch dog,
but didn't get no bed dog. Didn't want to give
up the quiet after Elbert's snoring stopped.
Some things about him I miss, but that's private.

Had these feelings I didn't know what to do with,
but then I remembered buryings. They are my chance
to give fleshly enjoyments a way out of the world.
I carry a foil-covered jar with plastic flowers,
set behind the family, and cry louder than Preacher.

Makes the kinfolks feel good to know a loved one
is getting a good grieving on his way to Paradise.
I let it out like a rocket going up at the fair.
What's wrong with that? Helps everybody feel better.
Livens up the show. Sometimes the undertaker smiles.

When the Lord opens his window and hollers for me,
I hope there's another healthy widow out there
looking for a place to lay out her black underwear.

The Present

Lori Russell

Min paused inside the door of the coffee shop and squinted at the pa-
trons. How would she find her daughter in this crowd? A wave of fear ran
through her. Then she heard Connie's voice and turned to see a blur of
blue waving in her direction from the far end of the restaurant.

"Hi, Mother," Connie said. "Did you find the place all right?"

"If I hadn't known it used to be Rosie's Donut Shop, I wouldn't have
recognized it. We came here every Saturday morning when you were
little."

"Chocolate old-fashioned donuts for the first sixteen years of my life. I
finally had to stop because I was getting pimples." Connie smiled. "The
place sure looks different doesn't it?"

Min looked around. The old red vinyl booths and the chrome-
trimmed counter were gone. The room smelled of coffee rather than cinnamon and fried dough. Min sat down on the metal seat of the chair. The
black wire bit into her flesh.

"They must not want anyone to linger too long. These chairs are terrible." Min sat forward to ease the pain in her back. "I can't stay long anyway. I have an appointment at ten."

"With the doctor? If you had told me earlier, I could have driven you."

"I'm only going across the street."

Connie looked out the window. "To the funeral parlor? Mother, you're
kidding."

"Yes, the funeral parlor. I figured it was time to make some arrangements."

A young woman appeared at Min's elbow. "Can I get you something
to drink?" she asked.

Min noticed the silver earrings hanging from the girl's ear. There were
at least six. One was a large cross. Min couldn't make out the others.

"I'd like a cup of coffee, please," she said.

"We have Sumatra blend, Colombian, or Indonesian." The earrings
rippled when the waitress moved her head.

"Coffee," Min said louder. The movement of the earrings must have affected the girl's hearing.

"Sumatra, Colombian, or Indonesian," the girl said again.

"Mother, those are kinds of coffee."

Min stared at Connie. This was so like her. Dragging Min to every new trendy restaurant in town regardless of what food they served.

"I just want a cup of coffee. Like the kind I make out of a can at home," Min said, staring at her daughter.

"Colombian," Connie said without turning to the waitress.

"Leaded or unleaded?"

"Leaded," Connie said. "And black."

Connie stretched her hands out on the table and began tapping the table with her freshly painted nails. "Now, what's this nonsense about," she paused and lowered her voice, "making funeral arrangements? Is it because of your birthday on Sunday?"

"Connie, I'm going to be seventy-eight. I'm way past the jumping-off point. I could go at any time." Min shifted in her chair. The hard seat was making her hip ache. "It's time I made some plans."

"But Mother, you aren't old. You're still getting out, still living on your own."

The waitress arrived with Min's coffee. "Anything else I can get you, ladies?"

"Thank you. That's all for now," Connie said sweetly. She turned to Min. "Mother, this talk about funerals is depressing. Let's talk about something more pleasant, like your birthday. Is there anything you need? A sweater? Maybe a colorful scarf?"

Accessories, the key to eternal youth, Min thought. She studied her daughter's outfit: a turquoise jogging suit with rhinestones and silver beads, pink and blue cacti hanging from her ears.

"Connie, I go out once a week with you for breakfast. Otherwise, I sit at home alone. I don't need anything. The only thing I want for my birthday is a coffin, and I'm going to take care of that this morning, myself."

"Mother!" Connie dropped her glass. A wave of brown liquid splashed onto the table. "See what you made me do!" Connie grabbed her napkin and began mopping.

Min stood slowly. A burning pain shot down her right leg. She held the edge of the table until it subsided then walked to the counter. "Could we have some napkins, please?" Min asked the waitress behind the register. "We had a small accident."

Min turned and watched Connie gather wet napkins and empty sugar packets. With a facelift and an auburn tint to cover the grey, her daughter looked much younger than her fifty-two years.

The waitress cleaned up the spilled coffee with two swipes of a rag. "Can I get you another *latte?*" she asked.

Connie waved her hands. "No, thanks." She put her fingers over the top of the glass. "I'm already a little jittery." After the waitress left, she leaned forward and smiled at Min. "Mother, where would you like to go for your birthday lunch?"

Min recognized that smile. Connie slipped it on like a warrior preparing for battle. "No gifts, no lunch. I've had enough birthdays in my life; I don't need to celebrate this one."

Connie's face pulled into a tighter smile. She took a bite of her bagel and swallowed carefully. "Nonsense, Mother. Every birthday is worth celebrating. There is a new place over on the water. I hear it has great seafood, and I know how much you like lobster."

Min slumped back into the chair and felt the chairback scrape her bones. "OK, Connie. Sunday for fish. Now I have to go." She gathered her purse and coat. "Thanks for the coffee."

Connie leaned over and kissed the air next to Min's cheek. "I'll pick you up at eleven on Sunday."

Outside, the weather was cooler than usual for October. A gust of wind swirled dry leaves around Min's ankles. She struggled to pull open the door at the funeral parlor, then felt the wind push her into the room as the door closed behind her.

"I'm Mrs. Minnetti," Min said to a dark-haired woman hunched over her computer. "I have an appointment."

"Of course, Mrs. Minnetti." The woman looked over the top of her glasses at Min. "Mr. Douglass will be right with you. Why don't you have a seat."

Min eased into a soft leather chair. The room wasn't the dark, dreary place she remembered when she visited after her husband, Sam's, death. The heavy, red chairs and flocked velvet wallpaper had been replaced by light-painted walls, a thick, grey carpet, and furniture the color of butter.

"Mrs. Minnetti? I'm Robert Douglass. It's good to meet you."

Min looked up and into eyes the same warm grey as the carpet. A thin man stood before her, hair cottony and thick, with silver-rimmed glasses perched on a long nose. When he smiled, his face exploded into a mass of lines. She had never seen wrinkles so beautiful.

"Please come with me," he said, directing her with a gentle touch of his hand on her elbow. His other arm hung limp in its coat sleeve.

Mr. Douglass's office was a large room with a pewter-and-gold patterned couch and two black overstuffed chairs. Min searched the pictures on the walls. These were not the stuffy oils usually found in offices, but colorful photographs of enormous towers covered with bright paper and flowers, black fabric bulls decorated with jewels. People with chocolate skin and dark hair carried platters of strange looking food. They were smiling.

"Ah, my photographs. Do you like them?" Mr. Douglass asked.

"They're very unusual," Min said, "and colorful. It looks like some kind of celebration."

"A Balinese cremation ceremony," said Mr. Douglass. "The villagers believe the soul is never free until there is a proper send-off. They parade the dead through the streets of the village on top of towers." He pointed to one of the photographs. "The bodies are then cremated inside those black bulls. Families spend years preparing. It's the greatest gift they can give their loved one."

"I wish Connie would take a trip to Bali," Min said, quietly.

"I beg your pardon?" Mr. Douglass reddened. "My hearing isn't what it used to be."

"I was just thinking about my daughter," Min said. "She didn't want me to come here today. She doesn't like the thought of me dying." Min smiled. "Or anyone else for that matter."

Mr. Douglass smiled and nodded.

"That's why I came to see you alone." Min straightened her shoulders and took a deep breath. "I want a blue one," she said firmly.

"A blue one?"

"Yes. A blue coffin. You see it's my favorite color. My entire house is blue. Outside, inside, all the furnishings. I just can't get enough of it." Min laughed. "I figure if I'm going to spend the rest of eternity in it, it will have to be blue." There. She had said it. Now there would be no confusing the issue, no trying to sell her something she didn't want.

Mr. Douglass smiled. "Well, of course. What a splendid way of putting it." He pulled a large, yellow tablet from his desk drawer. "And would that be a solid or split lid?"

"Split." She didn't want to have to worry about what shoes to wear or whether her stockings matched her dress.

"And what would you like for the interior?"

Min paused.

"We have satin, velvet, leather..."

"I hadn't really thought about it. Other than the outside, I mean. Can I look at some samples?"

The lines around Mr. Douglass's eyes crinkled. "Of course. We have a number of possibilities that might interest you. If not, we can special order."

Min followed him to the next room. It's like buying a new car or a sofa, she thought.

The room was large and softly lit. They walked past a row of undersized caskets. Min paused a moment, resting her hand on a white one with an angel carved in the lid. An old pain burned in her throat. "I lost a baby once," she said in a low voice. "It was back when they didn't have funeral services for stillborn babies."

"A girl or boy?"

"A little boy. Four years younger than my daughter. Connie was afraid to go to sleep for months afterward thinking she might die too." Min stroked the cheek of the angel with her thumb. "His name was going to be Andrew. I painted the nursery blue and put clouds on the ceiling." She smiled sadly and looked at Mr. Douglass. "Maybe that's why I love blue."

"I'm sorry, Mrs. Minnetti."

"No, I'm sorry." Min pulled her purse up on her shoulder. "I don't know what came over me. I haven't thought of that in years."

She continued walking past the coffins: dark mahogany with red satin lining, simple pine with beige velveteen, even steel grey with navy blue pinstripes.

Mr. Douglass rested his hand on a coffin that reminded Min of a Snickers bar: golden wood flecked and swirled with a darker richer brown.

"I thought you might like an interior in this color." He raised the lid to reveal a rich satin with just a blush of pink. "It would look beautiful with your skin."

Was it her imagination or did his eyes sparkle? Min ran her hand over the fabric. She was overcome with the urge to feel it against her face. "Can I try it? I mean... can I get inside?"

"Absolutely! I'm so glad you asked." He produced a small stool from under one of the coffins.

Min pulled her skirt up just above her knees and took Mr. Douglass's hand. She hadn't thought much about coffins until this week, let alone ever wanting to climb into one. But as she settled on the soft padding, getting into the casket seemed the most natural thing in the world.

"Go ahead. Lie down, Mrs. Minnetti. See how it feels."

Min stretched out on the thick cushion and rested her arms on her chest. The folds of satin surrounded her like a light hug.

"I must say, the pink does become you," said Mr. Douglass. He was smiling at her.

Min studied her hand against the satin. She never would have thought of pink. "Do you have a mirror?"

"Why Mrs. Minnetti, I believe you're the first to ever ask that. But yes, I think so. Let me ask my granddaughter."

In the stillness, Min felt the padding reach up and cradle her bony self. She closed her eyes. So this is how it will be. Not scary or suffocating. Comfortable. Quiet. Like so many of the hours she spent at home these days.

"So how is it?"

Min opened her eyes to find Mr. Douglass peering in at her.

"Wonderful."

"It's always good to take a test drive." He passed her a green hand mirror. "Makeup is included, if you're interested."

"Makeup?" Min studied her face. The pink did bring out a flush in her cheeks.

"Oh, yes. My granddaughter, Katherine, is studying to be a cosmetologist. She does a wonderful job. Families say their beloved often look more natural in death than they do in life."

"I haven't worn makeup in years." Min pictured her daughter peering into the open casket and seeing a pair of red lips. A mischievous thrill ran through her. She giggled. "I like the pink satin. Let me think about the makeup."

Mr. Douglass held out his hand and helped Min out of the casket. "Why don't we go back to my office and complete the paperwork. Would you like some tea?"

She watched him carry a gold-rimmed cup and saucer to the desk in his right hand, returning for a second set, and finally for the matching teapot. It was not the china nor the tremulous hand holding it that intrigued her. It was the man's other hand, hanging next to his body, its fingers curled stiffly in a lifeless palm. The skin was mottled, and dark branches of veins curved through tufts of black hair and disappeared under the jacket sleeve.

Sam, her husband, had died at fifty, slipping out of the world easily while asleep one night. He avoided watching death's slow approach, feeling the stiffness of age creep up his back and weigh heavily on his shoulders. He left Min to confront knobby knuckles and crepe skin alone.

Min watched Mr. Douglass pick up the motionless hand and place it in front of him on the desk. She looked up into his eyes.

"A stroke," he said, his mouth pulling up slightly at one corner. "Can't do a thing with the hand or the arm anymore. Just pack it around."

"You can't feel anything?" Min reached across the desk and grasped the clawed hand in hers. It felt cool.

Mr. Douglass shook his head.

It was as if he had one arm in the grave and life held the rest of him. Min flushed. Where was she coming up with these crazy thoughts?

"I'm sorry," Min whispered, and returned her hands to her lap. She felt hot and slightly giddy like she had had a glass of sherry.

Again she looked at the curled hand. "As the days pass, I seem to move farther and farther away. My body is getting slower and more clumsy, and I can't see well. So I go traveling. Not anywhere really. Just inside where it's quiet."

Mr. Douglass nodded. His eyes focused on her as she talked, unlike Connie's whose flitted about the room looking for something more comfortable on which to land. Min wanted to tell him more.

"Sometimes, I forget to eat. Just look at me. I've turned to skin and bones." She held out her arms to show him. "I stay inside myself more and more. It's like being halfway between awake and asleep. Peaceful. But then the telephone rings or some crazy commercial screams out of the TV, and I'm back here in the world again. One time," she leaned forward and whispered, "I was gone so long I even peed on myself." Min giggled. "I shouldn't tell you this, Mr. Douglass. My daughter won't even talk about it." Her voice became quiet. "I just thought you'd understand."

"I do. For me, death is the next big adventure." He pushed his glasses up his nose. "My bags are packed."

Min settled back into her chair. "You do understand."

"Mrs. . . . uh . . . may I call you Minerva?"

"Min. Please, call me Min." She felt sweaty again. She hadn't had hot flashes in years.

"I'm Robert." He smiled. "So many people come in here, pick out something quickly, then go home and try to forget about it. Or worse, they leave it to their families to take care of after they are gone. It's a pleasure having you here today."

"I just had to talk to someone about all of this." Min took a sip of tea and felt the liquid warm her chest.

"Do you know what you want for the service?"

"I know what I don't want. I don't want a minister that I don't know talking about me or an organ groaning in the background."

Robert laughed and waved a hand in front of his face. "Oh, no! Too medieval. People are doing all kinds of things these days: throwing ashes out of hot air balloons, having a wake at the zoo. It doesn't have to be tradition." His glasses had slipped to the end of his nose in his excitement. The flush of his skin made his eyes seem more blue than grey.

"Robert, I'll bet you have an incredible one planned."

"Actually," he paused to adjust his glasses, "I do. I want one of those old-time New Orleans jazz bands to lead a procession down the street. Women will be wearing magnolia blossoms on floppy hats, and there will be dancing in the streets. Two black horses will pull a buggy with me in a bright red casket. What a send-off!" Robert grinned, and his ears reddened. "Now Min, you have me talking about myself. What do you want?"

"Well, I like flowers. Peonies. My niece grows them in her garden: pink, white, as big as my hand." She spread her fingers wide to show him. "I've loved them since I was a child. I used to just stare at them, following the spiral of petals until I was in another world."

"How wonderful."

"Yes, but they don't grow well out here. The winters aren't cold enough. Oh, and roses, homegrown roses, not those sterile hothouse ones you get at the florist. I want scented ones." Min stopped. She hadn't talked this much in weeks. At home there were only the plants to talk with and occasionally a TV news commentator to yell at. Now here she was, words spilling out of her like a waterfall.

"There's a little white clapboard church up at Miller's Beach. Have you been there?"

The corners of Robert's mouth pulled into a soft smile. "Not in years."

"I just love it. Very simple. It would look great with all the flowers. My grandson, Ben, could play the music. Hammer dulcimer. His mother thinks it's crazy that he spends so much time with that instrument, but he plays it beautifully." She pointed to the yellow paper. "Put down 'Irish music,' he can pick which one, and 'On a Clear Day You Can See Forever.' That Barbra Streisand, I just love her."

Min waited while Robert slowly printed the information on the tablet. "Just make the rest simple. People can get up and say something if they wish. Afterward, I want a big party out on the beach. Oysters, clams, corn on the cob with lots of butter."

Min closed her eyes. She could see the day, warm and sunny. The church was beautiful, the flowers magnificent. It looked more like a party than a funeral. She felt an urge to pull off her shoes and dance on the beach, to lick the melted butter dripping from her fingers.

"Is there anything else I can do for you?" Robert was watching her.

"Yes, there is." Min sat up straight in her chair. "I'll be seventy-eight on Sunday. My daughter and I were going to have lunch at some new trendy restaurant, but I've changed my mind. Would you join us for corn on the cob and oysters at Miller's Beach?"

Robert nodded. "I'd be delighted."

Min signed the papers. "Thank you, Robert. You have made a difficult experience very enjoyable. I'll let you know about the makeup."

He held her hand for a moment, then released it.

Outside, the harshness of the wind had eased. The sun warmed Min's face. She walked down the block past a phone booth. I'll call Connie about the change of plans later, she thought. She opened the door to Kinney's Drugs and found her way to the cosmetics counter. Plucking a tube of lipstick from the display, she rounded her lips to an O and slid on the pink cream. It tasted a little like candle wax.

"May I help you?" a blond saleswoman asked from behind the counter.

"Yes," Min smiled. "I need some lipstick for a party on Sunday. It's my birthday."

The Lovers at Eighty

Marilyn Taylor

Fluted light from the window finds her
sleepless in the double bed, her eyes

measuring the chevron angle his knees make
under the coverlet. She is trying to recall

the last time they made love. It must have been
in shadows like these, the morning his hands

took their final tour along her shoulders and down
over the pearls of her vertebrae

to the cool dunes of her hips, his fingers
executing solemn little figures

of farewell. Strange—it's not so much
the long engagement as the disengagement

of their bodies that fills the hollow
curve of memory behind her eyes—

how the moist, lovestrung delicacy
with which they let each other go

had made a sound like taffeta
while decades flowed across them like a veil.

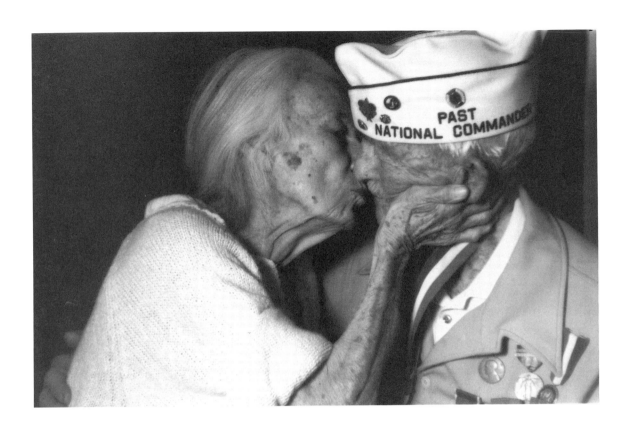

Blackberry Wine

Ruth Moose

The bed she died in
my grandfather never knew.
Summers she slept
in the front bedroom; white walled
and honeysuckle scented lace
curtains fingered by wind
from three tall windows.
She slept on feather pillows
plucked and filled by no hands
but hers.

That August, that
dry, dry August, she spent
in the place between dark and day,
sipping soup, cool tea, honey water,
cracked ice, and finally nothing
but blackberry wine. This teetotaler
who'd never touched whiskey nor
soda, drank her wine, told a risqué
joke, and laughed; this quiet woman
of the pious face, Victorian ways.
Grandmother told of an old maid,
a nun, and the man who came
in the night.

Death listened
found she was not afraid, took her hand.
At ninety-three she knew
she couldn't outbluff him,
so she went
calling her greeting ahead.

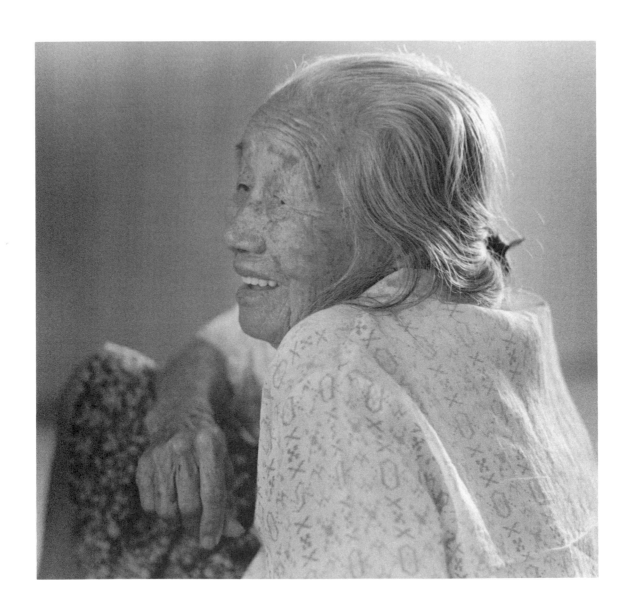

The Year Alice Moved to the Attic

Kathryn Etters Lovatt

"Did I ever tell you about that summer," she asked Clayton, "the one when I lived along New River?"

Alice's chair faced the window, but she knew her son stood an arm's length behind her, slightly bent under the threat of the roof's slant.

This attic was a hazard for anyone over five feet. In the last twenty years, she'd wasted by at least three inches, making the eaves and angles perfectly cozy as far as she was concerned. Clayton, on the other hand, would never fit up here, no matter how long he lived. He took a size twelve shoe before puberty.

"Enough, Mama," he scolded, discounting any story she intended to tell. "There's not a single comfort in this miserable space. Nothing anyone wants anymore." He brushed his hands together, as if to clean off cobwebs. "What on God's earth possesses you to sneak up here, to this dust and trash? You know it worries me sick."

Alice wasn't anxious to listen to what was coming. Steep steps and vertigo, how everyone else felt, she'd heard it so many times that she ignored Clayton now without much of a bad conscience. But he started with that nervous hack, and she didn't believe she could stand bad news just then.

"One year, my father rented a cottage for the entire season," she started again, quietly, hoping he'd lean in to hear. "Very small. Like a cabin. My mother refused anything to do with the place. Said it smelled like fish. I suppose it did, too. You either like that or you don't."

"I have no idea if you're eating, Mama."

Alice watched Clayton's hunchback shadow on her wall. It waved gnarly arms, shrugged padded shoulders.

"I have no idea if you remember to take your medicine; I don't know if you do take it and can't remember, and then you take some more." There was barely enough wind in him to finish. "No one's getting a bit of sleep," he told Alice, glad to have it out.

She wanted to assure him that she was, but she didn't think the soundness of her sleep counted for much. She wanted to tell about how she ended up here a little at a time, rambling through boxes, hunting letters she wrote once, but never mailed.

One search tired her so, she'd fallen dead to the world on the unmade bed. When she awoke, rested, she set the spot in order, liking its snug demands. She considered saying she found comfort here, and peace, but kept it to herself, fearing she might lose her story's place.

"I begged till my mother was glad to be rid of me and sent me on with my father. Every morning, Papa made that awful drive to the bank, and an old woman—not near as old as I am now—stayed the day with me. All we did was fish and nap and wade. Neither of us could swim a lick. Let me think, I'd turned seventeen that March. Mama sent me a ring with a blue stone, but I lost it that summer. Slid off my finger and down river, I guess."

When Clayton squatted behind her, she heard his knees crack. She even believed she heard the fabric of his dress pants shimmying up his calves, wondered if that rocking sound came with prayer or impatience. How extraordinary, she thought, the way senses narrow with age. Lately, her hearing seemed as selective as her memory.

Sometimes the simplest things eluded her: where the grandchildren lived, whose baby she'd rocked last Christmas, her telephone and social security numbers, her zip code. Many a day, she couldn't call the year itself. Often she misplaced remote details, but in this attic, everything important became close and obvious.

This morning, for instance, she admired lace around a pillowcase she pulled from a steamer trunk. Soon as she saw the delicacy of that border, she called her girlfriend's name. "Mary Lee Haskin," she said with absolute conviction. She could picture Mary tatting on the small shuttle, the eggshell lace edging the sallow muslin case, both white against the bright blue of Mary Lee's dress. Alice could hear her consumptive cough, too. That rasp paced the shortest of their walks until one damp night, while the two of them were doubled over one another laughing on the porch swing, Mary's breath began to slip away for good.

Alice felt sorrier for herself now than she ever had for her friend. How much more pathetic was this drawing out, this going beyond use.

Clayton squirmed behind her, rightly confused, she thought, at her sudden sniveling. He was a good son with something to say and no gift to say it. Bumbling and anxious, he wet his lips, but Alice made him wait.

"My little bedroom lay between two knuckles of that big river," she remembered, putting Mary away so completely she forgot Mary'd broken into her thoughts at all. "It was a miracle it survived there, perched out on a crook of sand, water creeping around like that."

Clayton had settled on a kidney-shaped footstool behind her. He smelled like an imported silk handkerchief.

"Oh, son," she said, "the lap of an inlet. It's some sound to live by." She wanted to look at him then, but didn't. He was never who she expected these days. "Sometimes, late at night, I think I hear it out there, still rippling under my window. I suppose it's my blood pressure though, or maybe my heart."

She patted her own cheeks then, which stung from remembering too much at once. Almost immediately that tingle made her realize what a mess she looked. Her hair, coarse and handsome when it first turned grey, had become baby fine and electrified these last few years. When she tried smoothing it now, the wisps crackled and stuck to her hands. Her partial plate floated in a pottery cup next to the oak bed; she hated that most.

Alice, who had slept in her duster and a cardigan, plucked a ball of maroon fuzz off the sweater's arm. Rolling the wool into a knot between her fingers, she recognized it was late morning at least, and Clayton ought to be at the bank.

"Surely it's not Saturday again?" she asked, twisting in her chair to see his reply. The pinched flush of his complexion surprised her more than his thin feathery hair or the wrinkles around the bow of his lip.

"Today is Tuesday," Clayton told her flatly. Before he could begin anything else, Alice was up, her cool dry forehead pressed against his.

"What is it, Mama, what are you doing?"

Alice would have sent him falling backward except for her claw-thin fingers gripping his temples. She was thinking it must be true, a nose never stops growing. She felt certain her own hooked more sharply today, at this very instant as she tried to keep it out of the way. She gave up and turned her wrist onto his brow. As she gauged Clayton's temperature, comparing it to her own, she wondered if her pulse was strong enough for him to feel.

"Have you been in the sun?" she asked, seeing his red splotched neck lump over his collar.

Clayton jerked up, leaving her empty-handed and still kneeling a little. She was sorry she said anything. He was overstarched from the beginning, she could see that from his stiff French cuffs. Now he was put out as well. He looked exactly as his father had when life fell off schedule. A fleshy sulk rose in his Irish cheeks; the jaw hinge clamped to a steely bluff.

Stooped over and pacing the unvarnished pine planks, Clayton stopped finally and shook his head at Alice. "We can't go on like this," he told her. "You know we can't."

Alice began making her way back to the window. She didn't sit right away. She watched two barrel-chested pigeons pecking shingle to shingle, and beyond that, she saw a mild sun split between two oaks. Her vision was too poor to spot a tulip poplar that had not bloomed these past three years.

"It's a blessing Ellie can drop in every day," Clayton told her. "But to find anybody for nights, that's something else again, Mama." Alice didn't move. "Ellie's not in any better shape than you are—why she's sixty-five if she's a day."

He pointed right at her while he went on—she thought she had taught him better than that—and seemed to grow larger with each word: a red balloon, inflating itself.

"She goes to pieces knowing you're up here and not answering," he said. "You'll kill yourself and her to boot before this is all over."

Alice could see how tiring this was for everyone. She was tired of it, too.

"I'm not afraid to stay alone," she promised.

Alice tried to understand how friends and family interpreted what she couldn't help. Had they convinced themselves that she stayed silent out of contrariness, that she would ignore Ellie or the phone ringing for the sake of pure meanness? The simple truth, which she didn't offer, was that she couldn't hear so well nowadays.

It occurred to Alice then: Little matter who came and went or sat or stayed the night, she was alone. No one knew her anymore.

Clayton prattled ambitiously in the background. "I've visited beautiful places, Mama. Places close by. You'll have your meals in a dining hall and play cards. Make friends. They have beauty parlors and greenhouses. They'll take you to the mall."

He was begging.

"Stop," she told him, and he did. She ached to the bone. A sour growl rolled through her stomach.

From the sky, Alice calculated noon, or close to it. "Come on," she said. "We'll fix lunch." She bobbed her bridge out of the cup and snapped it in.

Alice refused to go down the stairs first, hating to slow someone else. Clayton approved as she took each step carefully. When she reached near-bottom, a place that made her eye-to-eye with him, she said plainly, "I know what I can do."

They ate tuna salad on wilted lettuce, two olives each. They halved a honey bun. It was over the table Alice recognized Clayton's attempts to reason with her. His talk of portable phones and carpet up the attic steps, it gave her a little hope. She felt certain she had some time of her own yet, and it made her giddy.

She chattered about the summer she gutted fish, dug for worms. When the current was strong, she boasted, she used to blow kisses to boys rafting by.

"There was this one," Alice remembered. "Were we ever sweet on one another."

When Clayton hopped lightly off the back stoop, his own step like a boy's, she blew him a kiss, too. He stopped in his tracks, nearly snapped his fingers with his own sudden sense of discovery.

"You never lived by that river, did you?"

Alice felt flirtatious and sly. "Is it so hard to believe I've kept a secret?" she asked.

Clayton didn't let on he was convinced either way, but he'd come around to a good humor this afternoon, and she wanted him to hold on to it. Alice laughed.

"You and your tales, Mama. You ought to write a book of fables before you die."

Maybe she would, she told herself, taking the steps more slowly than ever. Her show of strength had tired her as much as trying to keep things straight. She would have liked to have told Clayton a story he wouldn't understand. And she wished she could explain this gradual shift, the slow attraction of sentiment.

In the attic finally, she drug a chamber pot from under her bed. She put out a tin of soda crackers. Everything back to its proper place, she curled in the dip of the only mattress that seemed to fit her bends and twists nowadays. She pulled a feather pillow, covered in Mary Lee's tatted case, toward her.

Alice drifted, a few shallow breaths on top of sleep, into a dreamy haze where she became a girl again, a girl of seventeen on a sunny afternoon. Perhaps it was Clayton Sr., younger than she ever knew him, who sat beside her on that rickety dock. As the old woman napped inside, perhaps he braided her hair with those dark, unlikely hands.

The hush-hush of water, the sound of his mouth on hers and his breath down her neck, the crush of her yellow cotton frock, she heard all of these rather than the doorbell. Every detail came with such clarity now, with such sweetness. Light caught the blue stone on Alice's finger; the river moved around her.

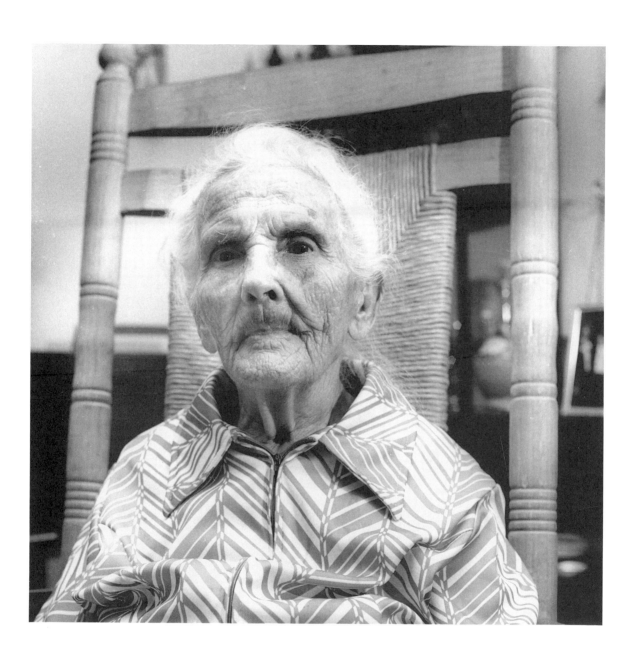

A Living Will

Naomi Halperin Spigle

When they say I cannot
hear you, sing me lullabies
and folk songs, the ones
I sang to you. I will hear them
as an unborn child can hear
its mother's music through
the waters of the womb.

When they say I can feel
nothing, press your face
against my forehead, rest your
hand against my cheek. I
will feel them as the woman
at the window feels the wind
outside the glass.

When they say I'm past
all caring, brush my hair
and braid in ribbons. I will
know it as the seashells
on my table know the
rhythms of the sea.

When they tell you
to go home, stay with me
if you can. Deep
inside I will be
weeping.

If Death Were a Woman

Ellen Kort

I'd want her to come for me smelling of cinnamon
wearing bright cotton   purple maybe   hot pink

a red bandana in her hair   She'd bring
good coffee   papaya juice   bouquet of sea grass

saltine crackers and a lottery ticket   We'd dip
our fingers into moist pouches of lady's slippers

crouch down to see how cabbages feel when wind
bumps against them in the garden   We'd walk

through Martin's woods   find the old house
its crumbling foundation strung with honeysuckle vines

and in the front yard   a surprise   jonquils
turning the air yellow   glistening and ripe

still blooming for a gardener long gone
We'd head for the beach wearing strings of shells

around our left ankles   laugh at their ticking
sounds   the measured beat that comes with dancing

on hard-packed sand   the applause of ocean and gulls
She'd play ocarina songs to a moon almost full

and I'd sing off-key   We'd glide and swoop
become confetti of leaf fall   all wings

floating on small whirlwinds   never once dreading
the heart-silenced drop   And when it was time

she would not bathe me   Instead we'd scrub the porch
pour leftover water on flowers   stand a long time

in sun and silence   then   holding hands
we'd pose for pictures   in the last light

Contributors

LIZ ABRAMS-MORLEY's poems have appeared in a variety of anthologies and journals including *Northeast Corridor, Nebraska Review,* and *Widener Review.* An inveterate people-watcher, trained family therapist, wife, daughter, and mother, she teaches at Community College of Philadelphia when not composing poems or carpooling, and works as an Artist-in-Residence in area public schools.

SARAH ALLEN is a sixty-two-year-old mother of four, grandmother of three, writer, internationally collected painter, and muralist with works in most of the States, Costa Rica, England, and Scotland. She is at work on three books.

KAYE BACHE-SNYDER explores inner and outer landscapes in writing and painting. Her poems appear in *Frogpond, Negative Capability, New Delta Review, Plainsongs,* and *Thema.* She enjoys hiking and bird-watching on mountains and prairies with her husband. With a Ph.D. in English and an M.A. in journalism, she teaches writing workshops for the University of Colorado-Boulder.

THERESE BECKER is a member of the National Press Photographer's Association. Her journalism and photojournalism have appeared in numerous newspapers, literary journals, and anthologies. She recently received her M.F.A. in Creative Writing from Warren Wilson College in Swannanoa, North Carolina. Her poetry has also been widely published, and she teaches workshops on the creative process throughout Michigan. She has recently combined her poetry and photography in a chapbook, *The Fear of Cameras.* ❧

TERRY BLACKHAWK has poems in numerous journals including *Iris, The Bridge, The Louisville Review,* and *College English,* and poetry awards from *America, The MacGuffin, Poetry Atlanta,* and *The Sow's Ear Review.* She enjoys teaching poetry to teenagers, but spent a wonderful sabbatical from that in 1992–93 as an NEH teacher-scholar studying Emily Dickinson.

JANE BLUE's work has appeared in many journals including *Ironwood, Carolina Quarterly,* and *The Prose Poem.* She has published two volumes of poetry, *The Madeleine Poems* (Trill Press, 1981) and *Sacrament* (Trill Press and Mt. Aukum Press, 1986). She received a master's degree in creative writing from U.C. Davis and has worked at a number of jobs, but recently she has devoted herself to a memoir, *My Mother and Amelia Earhart.* She has four grown children and three grandchildren and lives with her husband, Peter Rodman, in Sacramento.

BARBARA BOLZ is a freelance writer who lives in Bloomington, Indiana, with her partner, Kath Pennavaria, their young and active son, Adam, and two perpetually disgruntled cats. She is currently seeking a publisher for her book *I Got It!: A Workbook about Menstruation for Girls and Teenage Women.* ❧

JAYNE RELAFORD BROWN performs her writing and teaches college composition, literature, women's studies, and writing workshops part-time. She received an M.F.A. in creative writing from San Diego State University. Her writing has appeared in such periodicals as *The Minnesota Review, Hurricane Alice,* and *Common Lives/Lesbian Lives,* and in such anthologies as *Wanting Women, The Poetry of Sex, Dykescapes,* and *Silver-Tongued Sapphistry.* She is the mother of three grown children and lives with her partner of five years in the suburbs east of San Diego, where she loves to garden, cook, make paper, and write.

STEPHANY BROWN was born in Washington, D.C., and now lives in Flagstaff, Arizona, with her husband and three daughters. Her short stories have appeared in *Other Voices, A Room of One's Own, The Next Parish Over: A Collection of Irish-American Writing,* and other publications. ❧

KIM LY BUI-BURTON is a Vietnamese-American poet, librarian, and mother of two. Her work has appeared in the *Earth First! Journal, Footwork: The Patterson Literary Review, Leviathon,* and *The Squaw Review 1993.* She lives surrounded by books in a rose-covered Victorian five blocks from the Pacific Ocean, and composes poems while walking her dog, Emily Dickinson.

LORI BURKHALTER-LACKEY was born and educated in Los Angeles, California, completing her photographic training at Otis/Parsons Art Institute. Her photography has been exhibited in many California galleries and has been featured in numerous Papier-Mache Press books including *When I Am an Old Woman I Shall Wear Purple* and *If I Had My Life to Live Over I Would Pick More Daisies.* Lori lives in Los Angeles with her husband, David, and their three cats. ❧

GRACE BUTCHER is Professor Emeritus of English from Kent State University's Geauga Campus. Her most recent book, *Child, House, World,* brought her the Ohio Poet of the Year award in 1991. She has been competing in track for over forty years and has been U.S. half mile champion many times. ❧

ANNE M. CANDELARIA is the daughter of an Illinois farmer and a prairie artist. After earning a B.A. in English and an M.A. in Spanish Literature at the University of Illinois, she moved to California in 1961. She has one son, John, an actor. Recently retired from teaching to pursue a second career in writing, she has studied through the UCLA Writers' Program and other courses. She shares Philip Levine's admiration for the great Spanish poets.

LU CARTER resides in a small Nebraska community and works as a registered nurse. She started writing when she was eight and has never stopped. Her poems have previously been published in *The Nebraska English Counselor* and *The Western Journal of Medicine,* and by The Vermillion Literary Project and The National League for Nursing.

JUDY CLOUSTON is a writer and speaker who weaves poetry into every aspect of her life. She survived a 1978 stabbing which left her partially paralyzed, and acquired her gift for creating poetry from life's experience through her struggle to make the adjustments necessary to living as a paraplegic.

MARIL CRABTREE lives in Kansas City, Missouri, where she writes poetry, fiction, reviews, and articles, works as a mediator, and tries to live close to nature in an old "recycled" inner-city house. She won Honorable Mention for "Living the Green Life" in the 1994 *Passager* Poetry Contest. ❧

BRENDA CRANK called her mother and said that someone wanted another of her poems for an anthology, that she wrote because it fulfilled an inner need to express herself, and that *she* never knew that other people would want to read her work. Her mother said, "*I* knew that."

BARBARA CROOKER has published around five hundred poems in magazines such as *Yankee, The Christian Science Monitor,* and *Country Journal,* and five books— *Obbligato* (Linwood Publishers) is the latest. A recipient of three Pennsylvania Council on the Arts Fellowships in Literature, she lives with her husband and three children near an old apple orchard. ❧

PAMELA DITCHOFF's poetry and fiction has appeared in several literary publications. She has published two teaching texts with Interact Press: *Poetry: One, Two, Three* and *Lexigram Learns America's Capitals.* She resides in East Lansing, Michigan, and has recently completed her first novel. ❧

SUE DORO has been a labor and feminist writer for over thirty years. She relocated from Wisconsin to Oakland, California, in 1986 at the age of fifty. The mother of five, she is currently working for the U.S. Department of Labor and is the poetry editor of *Tradeswomen Magazine.* Her books include *Of Birds and Factories* (1983), *Heart, Home and Hard Hats* (Midwest Villages and Voices, 1986), and *Blue Collar Goodbyes* (Papier-Mache Press, 1992). ❧

SUSAN EISENBERG is a Boston-based writer, mother, union electrician, teacher, and activist/artist. She is currently touring a mixed media exhibit, *NOT on a SILVER PLATTER,* that uses poetry, stories, found objects, cookies, and soft sculpture to analyze federal affirmative action policies. She teaches theater workshops using historical monologues as scripts. ❧

LINDA NEMEC FOSTER is the author of three poetry chapbooks; the most recent is *Trying to Balance the Heart* (Sun Dog Press). Her poems have appeared in various publications including *The Georgia Review, Indiana Review, Nimrod,* and *Negative Capability.* She lives in Grand Rapids, Michigan, where she directs the literature program for the Urban Institute for Contemporary Arts.

AMY GEISHERT is a thirty-year-old lesbian feminist who is just starting to realize the importance of the visual in her life. She is striving to live more fully and more spiritually. She resides in Lansing, Michigan, with her partner and their two cats, Misha and Nickel. Oh yes, and she *loves* the color red!

MARIANNE GONTARZ is a social worker and a professional photographer, combining her work in such photography projects as the Boston Women's Health Collective's *Ourselves Growing Older.* Her photographs illustrate a number of professional books and journals in the field of aging including *A Consumer's Guide to Aging* (The Johns Hopkins University Press, 1992). She lives and works in Marin County, California. ❧

MAGGI ANN GRACE believes in the importance of the imagination and self-expression at all levels of the educational process. She teaches creative writing in schools, prisons, shelters, adult education programs, and through the Writer-in-the-Teacher Project for public school teachers. She holds an M.F.A. from UNC-Greensboro and now lives and writes in Chapel Hill, North Carolina. ❧

HARRIETTE HARTIGAN is a photographer, writer, teacher, and midwife. Her company, ARTEMIS, produced The Birth Disc, a laser disc of 10,000 images of the childbirth experience; publishes extensively; creates art prints and interactive visual presentations; and works with an international network/community of women making their lives visible.

SUSAN CAROL HAUSER is a poet and essayist. Her first book, *Meant to Be Read Out Loud*, received a 1989 Minnesota Book Award. Her other books include *Girl to Woman* and *Which Way to Look*. She holds an M.F.A. in poetry from Bowling Green State University, Ohio.

ANNDEE HOCHMAN is a freelance writer whose profiles, features, book reviews, essays, and short fiction have appeared recently in *Ms., Philadelphia* magazine, and *The Philadelphia Inquirer*. Her first book, *Everyday Acts & Small Subversions: Women Reinventing Family, Community, and Home*, was published in 1994 by The Eighth Mountain Press. She is pleased to report that she likes her nose; more importantly, she likes the face, body, and spirit that have grown up around it.

JUDITH INFANTE has an M.F.A. in Creative Writing from Vermont College and belongs to writing groups in San Antonio, Texas, and in Mexico City, D.V. Her poems have appeared in various anthologies and literary publications such as *High Plains Literary Review* and *American Poetry Review*. Her translations of contemporary Mexican poetry have been in *Manoa*, in anthologies from Four Winds Press, and in *El Tucan de Virginia*.

MARILYN JOHNSON teaches writing at California State University, Long Beach, and is one of the editors of *Pearl* literary magazine. Her poetry appears in an anthology, *A New Geography of Poets* (University of Arkansas Press), and her book, *A Necessary Fire*, was published in 1992 by Event Horizon Press.

ALLISON JOSEPH, a first generation Afro-Caribbean American, was born in London and raised in Toronto, Canada, and the Bronx, New York. Educated at Kenyon College and Indiana University, she is the author of *What Keeps Us Here*, a poetry collection that won the Ampersand Press Women Poets Series Competition in 1992. She is now an Assistant Professor of English at Southern Illinois University.

JUDE KEITH's work represents her approach to anti-bias imagery. The diversity of her subjects encourages the viewer to consider both political and human aspects of relationships and creativity. Combined with a strong commitment to children, her future work will include photography for children's picture books and textbooks. Her photographs have appeared in *If I Had My Life to Live Over I Would Pick More Daisies* (Papier-Mache Press, 1992) and several cards and small publications nationwide. ❧

MARY SUE KOEPPEL, editor of *Kalliope, a journal of women's art*, won the 1992 national Esme Bradberry Contemporary Poets Award from Wordart. Her poetry, fiction, and articles have appeared in over fifty publications including *Life on the Line* (Negative Capability), *Clockwatch Review,* and *Small Press Review. Writing— Resources . . .* (Prentice Hall) is her book of tips for emerging writers.

ELLEN KORT, who lives in Appleton, Wisconsin, has published five books of poetry and is a recipient of the Pablo Neruda Prize for Poetry. She has taught at the Oklahoma Summer Arts Institute at Quartz Mountain and the Rhinelander School of the Arts, and has traveled the U.S., Australia, New Zealand, and the Bahamas to present poetry readings and workshops ❧

MINDY KRONENBERG is a poet, writer, and teacher at Suffolk Community College whose work has appeared in over two hundred periodicals in the U.S. and abroad. In 1986 she was First Prize winner in the Chester H. Jones Foundation national poetry competition, and her work has been nominated for both the General Electric Younger Writer Award and the Pushcart Prize. She is the editor of *Book/Mark,* a small press review, and the author of *Dismantling the Playground,* a poetry collection.

KAY LOFTUS was born in El Cajon, California, in 1909. She came late to poetry writing at age seventy-five and has since had her haiku published in *Modern Haiku.* A retired teacher, she has had other poems appear in California retired teachers' publications. She frequently reads her poetry to groups in San Diego and North San Diego County, where she lives.

JEANNE LOHMANN lives in Olympia, Washington. Her work has appeared in many periodicals and in anthologies. She has published a prose memoir, *Gathering a Life* (John Daniel & Co., 1987), and four poetry collections: *Bonnie Jeanne* (with Harry A. Ackley), *Where the Field Goes, Steadying the Landscape,* and *Between Silence and Answer* (Pendle Hill, 1994). Originally from Ohio, she spent over thirty years in San Francisco, where she earned an M.A. in Creative Writing at San Francisco State University. She has four children and six grandchildren, sometimes wears purple, and enjoys doing readings and teaching poetry workshops.

JOYCE LOMBARD, Ventura, California, psychotherapist, specializes in issues of illness, loss and grief, and women's spirituality. She is coauthor of *Living Creatively with Chronic Illness* and *Joint Efforts: An Arthritis Movement Program.* Her poetry has recently appeared in *Art/Life, Rivertalk,* and *Verve.* She has begun a new business in handmade paper products, which includes limited edition books. Hiking and backpacking are photo and writing opportunities which show up in her work.

KATHRYN ETTERS LOVATT, a native of Camden, South Carolina, lives and writes in Jakarta, Indonesia. She has a masters degree in creative writing from Hollins College in Virginia and is a former fiction editor of Carolina Wren Press. Her work has most recently appeared in *The O. Henry Festival Stories* and *The Crescent Review.*

KATHARYN HOWD MACHAN, author of sixteen books, including *Belly Words* (Sometimes Y Publications), *Redwing Women* (CrazyQuilt Press), and *The Kitchen of Your Dreams* (Thorntree Press), and former director of the national Feminist Women's Writing Workshops, is also *Zajal*, professional belly dancer. With an M.A. in literature from the University of Iowa and a doctorate in performance studies from Northwestern University, she teaches writing at Ithaca College, and, with fellow poet Eric Machan Howd, is active as parent to CoraRose and Benjamin. ❦

CHRIS MANDELL, thirty-five, lives in Boston where she teaches elementary art and plays acoustic and electric violin. She hopes that her poem, "A Place to Rest," might give strength and hope to anyone trying to recover from an eating disorder. She dedicates this poem to Dr. Jerome Bass who has been instrumental in helping her find a firmer place to rest.

BILLIE BARBARA MASTEN, mountain woman and poet performer, lives on the apron of the coastal mountains in Big Sur, California. She wrote *Owning the Beast and the Bad Girl* to start acknowledging her dark side. She has also published *Billie Beethoven* and *His & Hers: A Voyage Through the Middle-Age Crazies*, the latter coauthored with poet Ric Masten, her husband of forty-two years. Now a crone, she leads ceremonies to celebrate being an elder.

BARBARA J. MAYER of Mooresville, North Carolina, is a former Chicago journalist whose poems have appeared in numerous publications including *Spoon River Quarterly*, *Iowa Woman*, and *Filtered Images: Women Remembering Their Grandmothers*. She has received the Sam Ragan Award from *Crucible* and the Archibald Rutledge Award from the Poetry Society of South Carolina.

JOANNE MCCARTHY writes and teaches in Tacoma, Washington. One of her poems crisscrosses Seattle on the Poetry Bus. More than ninety others have appeared in anthologies and magazines including *Poets On:*, *Green Fuse*, and *The Bellingham Review*. She loves Reese's peanut butter cups and has just learned to swim. ❦

MARY MCGINNIS has lived, written, and worked in New Mexico since 1972. The empty places of the desert and the edges of cliffs have changed her poetry into more direct expressions of tenderness, anger, and delight. She has given poetry readings at various bookstores and galleries in Philadelphia, Albuquerque, Taos, and Santa Fe. A feminist and disability rights activist, she trains peer counselors at an independent living center and also counsels people with disabilities. Her two great loves are writing poetry and counseling. She published a chapbook, *Private Stories on Demand*, in 1988 and is currently working on another chapbook.

SHIRLEY VOGLER MEISTER is an Indianapolis freelance writer whose prose and poetry appears in diverse U.S. and Canadian publications. She has earned awards for poetry, journalism, and literary criticism. Her poem, "The Coming of Winter," is in *When I Am an Old Woman I Shall Wear Purple* (Papier-Mache Press, 1987); another, "The Sacrifice," is in *If I Had My Life to Live Over I Would Pick More Daisies* (Papier-Mache Press, 1992). ❦

ANN MENEBROKER was born in Washington, D.C., and has lived in Sacramento for forty years. She is an assistant at an art gallery and on the board of the Sacramento Poetry Center. She has published poems in various journals including *Caprice, Bogg,* and *Painted Bride Quarterly.* She is also a finalist judge for *Pearl's* chapbook contest in fall 1994. Her most recently published collections include *Routines That Will Kill You* (Bogg Press, 1990), *Mailbox Boogie, A Dialogue Through the Mails* (Zerx Press, 1991) with Kell Robertson, and *Dream Catcher* (Red Cedar Press, 1992). ❧

S. MINANEL, due to some right-brained activity, has had her graphics and doggerel published in periodicals such as *Redbook, Light, Personal Computer Age, AB Bookman's Weekly, Sky & Telescope, Sailing, Pacific Yachting, Ensign, Young American, Computeredge,* and *Beverly Hills, The Magazine.* She is still waiting to hear from her left brain. ❧

MICHELE MOORE earned a degree in Physical Therapy from Georgia State University and an M.F.A. in Writing from Vermont College. Her short fiction has appeared in *ACM (Another Chicago Magazine), The Habersham Review,* and *Groundwater,* and is forthcoming in *The Louisville Review.* She has received grants for fiction writing from the Kentucky Foundation for Women and the Kentucky Arts Council. Her physical therapy goals are always about movement: increase it, make it safer, make it hurt less. Her fiction goal is also about movement: increase it, take more risks, make it hurt . . . less?

RUTH MOOSE has published in *Atlantic Monthly, Redbook, Ladies' Home Journal, Yankee,* and other places. She is the author of two books of short stories: *The Wreath Ribbon Quilt* and *Dreaming in Color* (August House). She lives in Albemarle, North Carolina, and teaches at Pfeiffer College.

LILLIAN MORRISON is the author of seven collections of her own poems, most recently *Whistling the Morning In* (Boyds Mills Press); three anthologies of poems on sports and rhythm including *Rhythm Road* (Lothrop) and *At the Crack of the Bat* (Hyperion); and six collections of folk rhymes for children. *Slam Dunk,* an anthology of basketball poems, is forthcoming from Hyperion. ❧

MARNIE MUELLER's first novel, *Green Fires: A Novel of the Ecuadorian Rainforest,* was published in 1994 by Curbstone Press. Her stories and poems have appeared widely, including in *Quarterly West, The Laurel Review, River Styx,* and the *Village Voice's VLS.* She is working on a novel set in the Tule Lake Japanese Internment Camp where she was born. ❧

SHARON H. NELSON works as an editor in Montreal, where she cooks and gardens seasonally. Her eighth book of poems, *Family Scandals* (The Muses' Company, 1994), follows *The Work of Our Hands* and *Grasping Men's Metaphors* in a series that explores the constructions of sexuality, language, and gender.

CAROL NEWMAN, a poet and writer, grew up in southwest Oklahoma among women who rode, roped, drove wheat trucks, and ran off with older men and returned telling tales of faraway places. It is from these women and for these women that Carol writes. She is now developing Caddo Creek, an eastern Kansas retreat for writers. She has recently completed her first novel, a mystery titled *In the Event of Death.*

LAURA APOL OBBINK is a poet and freelance writer whose work has appeared in a number of journals and periodicals. She recently completed a Ph.D. at the University of Iowa and lives with her family in Norman, Oklahoma.

MAUREEN O'BRIEN teaches writing and literature at St. Joseph College in West Hartford, Connecticut. Her work has appeared in *Hurricane Alice, Kalliope,* and other publications and was recognized in the 1992 World's Best Short Short Story Contest. She lives in central Connecticut with her husband, Tim, and her children, Madeline and Max.

KEDDY ANN OUTLAW writes fiction, poetry, and book reviews. Her work has appeared in the *1989 Houston Poetry Fest Anthology, Exit 13, Perceptions, Karamu, i.e. magazine, Library Journal,* and the *Houston Chronicle.* She works as a branch librarian for the Harris County Public Library System in Houston, Texas.

KATHY M. PARKMAN was born in Fresno, California, and lived there for twenty-four of her twenty-seven years. She received her M.F.A. in creative writing from Mills College in 1993. Her short "autobiografiction" often focuses on women and the bodies they live in.

KATHLEEN PATRICK is a poet and fiction writer whose work has appeared in many literary magazines and anthologies. Her poetry has received several awards including a Loft-McKnight Award and a recent Jerome Travel Grant to continue work on a new collection of poetry. She lives in Minnesota with her family.

ANNA PRICE-ONEGLIA is a Monterey Bay Area painter who was born in New York City. She made the cover image with transparent watercolor and Japanese paper.

SANDRA REDDING is an M.F.A. graduate of the University of North Carolina-Greensboro and teaches creative writing at local colleges. She's published over twenty short stories. Her story published in *When I Am an Old Woman I Shall Wear Purple* (Papier-Mache Press, 1987) has been incorporated into a play, *Pitstop,* currently touring the South. She's now working on a novel based on the characters in the story she published in *If I Had My Life to Live Over I Would Pick More Daisies* (Papier-Mache Press, 1992). ❧

BERNICE RENDRICK has lived in California most of her life but was born in Kansas. She returned to school at midlife, discovered poetry, and has since published in numerous journals and anthologies. She is a member of the Santa Cruz Writers' Union and the California State Poetry Society. Her long friendship with Joan Savo was a source of inspiration and encouragement that continues through paintings, letters, and memories. ❧

ANNE GILES RIMBEY is a columnist for the Tampa Bay Area creative writing newsletter, *Plexus.* She received an Emerging Artists Grant for poetry from the Arts Council of Hillsborough County, Florida. Her work has appeared in *New Voices* and other magazines.

MARIE KENNEDY ROBINS depicts humor as well as tragedy in the patois of rural women of the South. Considered by some to be a new art form, her prose poems were featured in an hour-long interview on WPFW-FM in Washington, D.C. She has had twenty poems published by St. Andrews Press. ❧

ROSALY DEMAIOS ROFFMAN is coeditor of the prize-winning *Life on the Line: Selection on Words and Healing*, and author of a poetry collection, *Going to Bed Whole*. She has read her poetry at two World Congresses of Poets in Israel and Mexico, and has been published nationally in journals, magazines, and anthologies. She collaborated with composers and a dance company on three different pieces that premiered nationally. Currently at Indiana University of Pennsylvania, she teaches writing, myth, and literature. She is presently working on a book on Orwell's poems, and on translations of Ladino poetry (with a grant from the Witter-Bynner Foundation).

ELAINE ROTHMAN spent twenty years as an educator. Upon retirement she freelanced as a feature story writer for Connecticut newspapers. Her fascination with ancient history led her to write a novel about the Etruscans. Whenever possible she joins naturalists' tours, traveling twice to Costa Rica, the setting for her latest fiction work. ❧

LORI RUSSELL is a freelance writer and public relations consultant. Her short stories have appeared in *If I Had My Life to Live Over I Would Pick More Daisies* (Papier-Mache Press, 1992), *Calyx*, and numerous literary journals. She lives with her husband and son in The Dalles, Oregon. ❧

JANE SCHAPIRO's poems have been published in literary journals such as *The American Scholar*, *The Gettysburg Review*, and *Poetry East*, as well as nonliterary journals such as *Journal of American Medical Association* and *Moment*. She is a freelance writer for *Bread for the City*, a Washington, D.C., food and medical program for the poor. She lives with her husband and three daughters in Fairfax, Virginia.

HEIDI SCHWEITZER, a resident of Waukesha, Wisconsin, recently received her B.A. in English from Carroll College. She is a photographer, writer, and bookseller for Harry W. Schwartz Bookshop. Her photography and poetry have appeared in *Century Magazine*. She would like to thank her mother, Helen, for her assistance with the self-portrait entitled "Joy" that appears in this anthology.

JAN EPTON SEALE is a poet and fiction writer from the Rio Grande Valley of Texas. Her publications include three books of poetry, nine children's books (Knowing Press and Houghton-Mifflin), a couple of produced plays, and a book of short stories, *Airlift*, published by T.C.U. Press. Seven of her stories have appeared in PEN Syndicated Fiction Projects over the years, two of them on National Public Radio. ❧

DEBORAH SHOUSE often feels a restless dissatisfaction with reality. So she creates fiction. Sometimes she feels a fondness for certain versions of reality. So she creates essays. Her work has appeared in *Christian Science Monitor*, *The Sun*, and *Tikkun*. She has a petite book of fiction, *White Bread Love*, and is coauthor of *Working Woman's Communications Survival Guide*.

ANITA SKEEN is Professor of English at Michigan State University where she teaches in the creative writing, women's studies, and Canadian literature programs. She is the author of two volumes of poems, *Each Hand a Map* and *Portraits,* and is currently working on a collection of fictional pieces. ♣

NAOMI HALPERIN SPIGLE was first published at the age of seven in her school newspaper. Sixty years later she dares to hope her writing has progressed. Her poems have appeared in four anthologies and two dozen literary journals, most recently *Kalliope, South Coast Poetry Journal, Fiddlehead,* and *Sifrut.* In 1992 she received an Indiana Individual Artist Fellowship.

AMBER COVERDALE SUMRALL has edited ten collections of writings by women, including *Catholic Girls, Lovers, Breaking Up Is Hard to Do,* and *Women of the 14th Moon: Writings on Menopause.* Her poetry has appeared in *Women's Review of Books, Pearl, Mid-American Review,* and *Negative Capability.* She is currently having a love affair with her bicycle.

CHRISTINE SWANBERG is the author of four books of poetry: *Tonight on This Late Road* (Erie Street Press, 1984), *Invisible String* (Erie Street Press, 1990), *Bread Upon the Waters* (Windfall Prophets Press, 1990), and *Slow Miracle* (Lake Shore Publishing, 1992). In 1994, Snapshot Music released a cassette of her poetry with piano, *Live on Route 2.* She has won various prizes including the YWCA Blanche Starr Award for the Arts, the C. Hall Connor Award for Fiction, and the grand prize from *Midwest Poetry.* She is public relations director at Rockford Business College. ♣

TERESA TAMURA, a photographer at the *Seattle Times,* is a native of Nampa, Idaho. After leaving her home state in 1989 to pursue her career, she has worked for the *Los Angeles Times* and the *Morning Call* in Allentown, Pennsylvania. She will begin her M.F.A. studies in photography at the University of Washington this fall while continuing to work part-time.

MARILYN TAYLOR teaches at the University of Wisconsin-Milwaukee, and is the author of a book of poems, *Shadows Like These* (Wm. Caxton, 1994). Her poetry has appeared in *Poetry, Poetry Northwest,* and a number of other literary journals and anthologies. She has recently received awards from the Associated Writing Programs and the Wisconsin Arts Board.

KATIE UTTER, a photographer/travel agent living near the ocean in Rhode Island, discovered her love of black-and-white photography at Hollins College in Virginia. Since then, she has studied photography at Syracuse University in London and at Connecticut College in New London, Connecticut. She perfects that love today, photographing young musicians studying string instruments using the Suzuki method.

AMY UYEMATSU is a Sansei (third generation Japanese-American) from Los Angeles. Her first book, *30 Miles from J-Town,* won the 1992 Nicholas Roerich Poetry Prize.

CLAUDIA VAN GERVEN lives in Boulder, Colorado, where she teaches writing. She has been published in various small magazines including *Prairie Schooner,*

Calyx, and *Sing Heavenly Muse.* She has works in several anthologies including *If I Had My Life to Live Over I Would Pick More Daisies* (Papier-Mache Press, 1992). She won the 1992 Russell Leavitt Memorial Award for poetry from the Florida State Poets Association. ❧

BEVERLY VOLDSETH publishes *RAG MAG* and is a secretary, teacher, newspaper columnist, grandmother, and lover of all things sensual. Rocks, tree bark, feathers, bleached animal bones, and skinny dipping are high on her list. Words are her most constant love affair. Each time they gather on the page, she is amazed by what they say.

ELIZABETH WEBER teaches creative writing at the University of Indianapolis. She has an M.F.A. from the University of Montana. Her poetry book, *Small Mercies,* was published by Owl Creek Press. Her poems have appeared in various magazines including *Calyx, Graham House Review, Puerto del Sol,* and *Iowa Woman.*

SUELLEN WEDMORE grew up in the Midwestern states of Illinois, Indiana, Ohio, and Wisconsin, but now lives and works as a speech and language therapist in picturesque Rockport, Massachusetts. She was fortunate to be awarded a sabbatical leave of absence for the 1993–94 school year so that she could pursue her love of writing.

ALISA WOLF is a freelance writer and editor who lives in West Medford, Massachusetts. She has helped edit and produce two community newspapers, an astronomy magazine, and other publications. Her work has been published in *Sojourner's* "First Person" column. She coparents a cat, Dino, who was born prematurely grey.

MICHELE WOLF's poems have appeared in *Poetry, The Hudson Review, The Antioch Review, Southern Poetry Review,* and many other literary journals and anthologies, including Papier-Mache's *When I Am an Old Woman I Shall Wear Purple* and *If I Had a Hammer: Women's Work.* She lives in New York, where she works as a magazine writer. ❧

MARY ZEPPA's poems have appeared in various publications including *Shaman's Drum, Zone 3, The New York Quarterly, Visions International,* and *Mixed Voices: Contemporary Poems About Music.* She is an associate editor of *Tule Review,* and is also a singer and lyricist. *Landing Signals, An Anthology of Sacramento Poets* includes both her poems and her song, "Lost Woman Blues." She is one-fifth of Cherry Fizz, an a cappella quintet specializing in doo-wop.

MARILYN ZUCKERMAN has published three books of poetry: *Personal Effects* (Alice James Books, 1976) with Helena Minton and Robin Becker, *Monday Morning Movie* (Street Editions), and *Poems of the Sixth Decade* (Garden Street Press, 1993). Her poems have also appeared in magazines such as the *New York Quarterly, Nimrod, The Little Magazine,* and *Pig Iron.* She had two poems published in *Ourselves Growing Older* from the Boston Women's Health Collective (Simon and Schuster, 1987) and a short story in the anthology *Word of Mouth 2* (Crossing Press, 1991). She has also received a 1985 PEN Syndicated Fiction Award.

❧ Denotes contributors whose work has appeared in previous Papier-Mache Press anthologies.

Acknowledgments

Grateful acknowledgment is made to the following publications which first published or accepted for publication some of the material in this book:

Negative Capability, Vol. 6, No. 4, Fall 1986 for "Before Stillbirth" by Barbara Bolz; *Silver-Tongued Sapphistry* (Silver-Tongued Sapphists Press, 1988) for "Finding Her Here" by Jayne Relaford Brown; *Room of One's Own*, Vol. 16., No. 4, December 1993 (The Growing Room Collective) for "Matchmaking" by Stephany Brown; *Beginnings, Endings and Somewhere-in-Between* (Potpourri Press, 1992) for "To My Body" by Judy Clouston; *West Branch*, Issue 11, 1982 and *The Lost Children* (The Heyeck Press, 1989) for "Applewood" by Barbara Crooker; *Heart, Home and Hard Hats* (Midwest Villages and Voices, 1986) and *Each in Her Own Way—Women Writing on Menopause* (Queen of Swords Press, 1994) for "Menopause Poem" by Sue Doro; *In Celebration of Babies* (Ballantine Books, 1987) for "Breastfeeding at Night" by Susan Eisenberg; *A History of the Body* (Coffee House Press, 1987) for "History of the Body" by Linda Nemec Foster; *Inside Magazine*, Spring 1993, for "What I Know from Noses" by Anndee Hochman; *A Necessary Fire* (Event Horizon Press, 1992) and *Pearl*, No. 3, Winter 1974 for "Womansong" by Marilyn Johnson; *If Death Were a Woman* (Fox Print, Inc., 1994) for "If Death Were a Woman" by Ellen Kort; *Spindrift*, Vol. 27, 1989 for "Plastic Surgery" by Mindy Kronenberg; *The New Hearer*, Vol. 1, No. 2, Jan./Feb. 1981 and *Steadying the Landscape*, 1982 for "Hearing" by Jeanne Lohmann; *Belly Words* (Sometimes Y Publications, 1994) and *Jareeda*, February 1994 for "Belly" by Katharyn Howd Machan; *Mediphors*, Spring 1994, No. 3, for "The Fat Lady Speaks" by Joanne McCarthy; *Wormwood Review*, Vol. II, #2, Summer and *Biting Through the Spine* (The Sacramento Poetry Exchange, 1985) for "This" by Ann Menebroker; *Art:Mag* (Limited Editions Press, 1988) for "The Naked Truth" by S. Minanel; *Christian Century*, Vol. 108, No. 24, 1991 for "Blackberry Wine" by Ruth Moose; *The Sidewalk Racer and Other Poems of Sports of Motion* (Lothrop, Lee and Shepard, 1977) and *Atalanta* (Papier-Mache Press, 1984) for "The Spearthrower" by Lillian Morrison; *The Work of Our Hands* (The Muses' Company, 1992) for "Premenstrual Syndrome" by Sharon H. Nelson; *Live Writers! Local on Tap*, Vol. 1, No. 2, 1980 (La Reina Press) for "Butchering Time" (previously "Cora's Vision") by Carol Newman; *Lilith*, Vol. 14, No. 4, Fall 1989 for "Tapping a Stone" by Jane Schapiro; *Conditions*, No. 15 for "Crossing the High Country" by Amber Coverdale Sumrall; *Indiana Review*, 14.3, 1991 and *Shadows Like These* (Wm. Caxton, 1994) for "The Lovers at Eighty" by Marilyn Taylor; *West/World 3*, Winter 1990–91 for "To Women Who Sleep Alone" by Amy Uyematsu; *Crone Chronicles*, No. 19, Spring 1994 for "Crone Drives through Spring" by Claudia Van Gerven; *Ophelia's Pale Lilies*, Vol. 1, Issue 7, 1990 for "After Reading Mark Strand's 'Courtship'" by Beverly Voldseth; and *Ourselves Growing Older* (Simon & Schuster, 1987/1984), *Only Morning in Her Shoes* (Utah State University Press, 1990), *Mother's Underground*, Issue 12, 1993, and *Poems of the Sixth Decade* (Garden St. Press, 1993) for "After Sixty" by Marilyn Zuckerman.

Papier-Mache Press

At Papier-Mache Press, it is our goal to identify and successfully present important social issues through enduring works of beauty, grace, and strength. Through our work we hope to encourage empathy and respect among diverse communities, creating a bridge of understanding between the mainstream audience and those who might not otherwise be heard.

We appreciate you, our customer, and strive to earn your continued support. We also value the role of the bookseller in achieving our goals. We are especially grateful to the many independent booksellers whose presence ensures a continuing diversity of opinion, information, and literature in our communities. We encourage you to support these bookstores with your patronage.

We publish many fine books about women's experiences. We also produce lovely posters and T-shirts that complement our anthologies. Please ask your local bookstore which Papier-Mache items they carry. To receive our complete catalog, send a self-addressed stamped envelope to Papier-Mache Press, 135 Aviation Way, #14, Watsonville, CA 95076, or call our toll-free number, 800-927-5913.